Health and Social Care: Knowledge and Skills

# Understanding Research and Evidence-based Practice

Health and Social Care: Knowledge and Skills

# Understanding Research and Evidence-based Practice

Bruce Lindsay

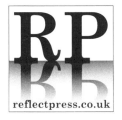

reflectpress.co.uk

First published in 2007

ISBN: 978 1 906052 01 0

**British Library Cataloguing in Publication Data**
A catalogue record for this book is available from the British Library

Production project management by Deer Park Productions, Tavistock, Devon

Typeset by Pantek Arts Ltd, Maidstone, Kent

Cover design by Oxmed

Printed and bound by Bell & Bain Ltd, Glasgow

Distributed by BEBC, Albion Close, Parkstone, Poole, Dorset BH12 3LL

www.reflectpress.co.uk

Published by Reflect Press Ltd
11 Attwyll Avenue
Exeter
Devon
EX2 5HN
UK
01392 204400

# Contents

# Author biography

Dr Bruce Lindsay is currently Deputy Director of the Nursing and Midwifery Research Unit, Faculty of Health, University of East Anglia.

Dr Lindsay has a special interest in systematic review of health care delivery and is the co-author of four reviews for the Cochrane Collaboration. He has undertaken research into a range of health and social care activities, particularly in relation to child health, nursing and the development of hospital care for children. He has also studied the use of randomised controlled trials in the assessment of complex health care interventions. In his research Dr Lindsay has used a wide range of methods, including systematic review, documentary analysis, surveys, interviews and observational studies. He also teaches research methods and research appraisal, and supervises postgraduate research students at masters and doctoral levels.

# Introduction

In a country such as the United Kingdom, health and social services employ large numbers of people, cost billions of pounds each year and can be found in almost every community, however small. Most colleges and universities offer courses for students hoping to work in health or social services. There are many different health and social care professions, with many practitioners.

Health and social care practice is the result of many factors. Some of it is controlled directly by government legislation. Some practice is controlled by local policies and procedures developed by individual companies, social service departments or National Health Service Trusts. Yet more practice is the result of custom, of having been done for so long that no-one can remember why. In contemporary health and social care, however, it is crucial that all practice is 'evidence based': that it can be justified by referring to some sort of reliable information or data. Much of the evidence for practice, though not all of it, comes from research. In other words, it comes from organised and deliberate investigations which result in the creation of information that can be applied to the organisation and delivery of care. 'Research' and 'evidence-based practice' are therefore vital concepts to understand if you want to understand health and social care practice.

This book aims to help you gain this understanding of research and evidence-based practice. I hope that in doing so it will help you to better understand your own practice and to develop skills that will enable you to become a valuable health or social care professional yourself.

## THE SCOPE OF THIS BOOK

This book will not turn you into a researcher, but I hope that it will help you to become an effective user of research findings and other evidence by helping you to understand what research is, how it's done, what it can and can't tell us and how it can provide evidence for practice.

Part One aims to make sense of the research process: the steps through which any researcher goes to develop, carry out and report on a research project. Each chapter focuses on one or two steps of this process, from the first ideas about what to study to the ways in which researchers make their work available to others.

Part Two concentrates on using evidence to inform practice. It discusses ways in which you can judge the usefulness of evidence for practice, how you can use it to inform your own practice and how it can be used to influence practice on a national or even global scale. Chapter 10 looks at ways of ensuring practice quality through audit and evaluation and compares audit and evaluation with research.

The final chapter looks at the future of research and evidence-based practice in health and social care. Much of this discussion focuses on possible developments in the short to medium term, when many readers of this book will be in their early professional careers. How will research and other evidence affect the ways in which your careers will develop and the environments in which you may practise?

## HOW YOU SHOULD USE THIS BOOK

You should, of course, read it. It's relatively short, for a textbook, so you could read it from cover to cover without too much difficulty. However, you don't have to read it all from start to finish. Each chapter is self-contained and can be read usefully on its own. Indeed, in order to fit your study needs most effectively it is likely that you will want to read some chapters more than others, or that you will read the chapters in a different order from the one in which they are presented.

Each chapter has features which will, I hope, make the book more interesting and make your learning more effective. I've called them 'keys' as they are intended to unlock ideas, to enable you to enter new areas of knowledge, or to act as important clues to help you solve problems.

***Key questions*** These appear at various points in each chapter, when there are important issues that you need to ask yourself about. Key questions do not necessarily have 'right' or 'wrong' answers and, indeed, in many cases you may not decide on an answer at all. They are brief exercises or hints for reflection which you should use to clarify your own ideas and understanding of research or evidence-based practice.

***Key cases*** These are short descriptions of real research studies, research activities, care activities or documents which help to illustrate crucial topics within the text.

*Key learning points* These appear at the end of each chapter and summarise the most important points. You should feel confident that you understand each key learning point before you move on.

In addition to the keys each chapter closes with a list of further reading. The lists are not intended to be exhaustive, but to offer you some recommendations for more detailed information. In most cases the choices should be self-explanatory, but where I have included a work that is not obviously related to the chapter I give a brief explanation for my choice.

Researchers and policy-makers seem to enjoy using jargon and it is impossible to write a book on research and evidence-based practice without repeating at least some of it. To help you understand this jargon, throughout the book you will find some words or phrases printed in bold **like this**. These terms are defined in the glossary located near the end of the book.

An understanding of two terms in particular is crucial to your use of this book: 'research' and 'evidence-based practice'. I've used both terms a few times already, but what do I mean by them?

## WHAT IS RESEARCH?

When people use the word 'research' they can do so in two major ways. There is the idea of research as an activity: 'I'm doing research' or 'I'm researching'. There is also the idea of research as a product: 'we're using research' or 'the research tells us to work like this'. In the latter case I think it is more correct to talk about research findings or results, not just research. In this book, when I refer to the products or outputs of research projects I will usually use the term 'research findings'. Research as a process or activity needs more careful consideration.

### Key Question 1

I want to know how tall the average resident of Britain is. I ask all my friends (62 people) how tall they are, then add up their heights and divide by 62. I decide that the answer tells me how tall the average resident of Britain is.

- Have I just done some research?
- Am I right to think that my result answers my question?
- If not, what should I have done?

Research, like many terms in health and social care, doesn't have a single definition that everyone agrees on. Some authors refer to research as systematic inquiry or structured investigation. Others emphasise the need for a question to be answered or a phenomenon or event to be explored or investigated. Some definitions are very short. The 2001 Research Assessment Exercise, carried out in higher education institutions in the UK, defined research briefly as '... original investigation undertaken in order to gain knowledge and understanding' (HERO, 1999, section 1.12). Burns and Grove (1999, p.3) define research as 'diligent, systematic inquiry or study to validate and refine existing knowledge and develop new knowledge'. Both of these definitions seem suitable to me. It is possible to find other, more complex, definitions but we need not get too complicated.

## The research process

The movement through the individual stages of a research project, from the initial idea to the communication of your findings to the wider world, is referred to as the 'research process'. Figure 1 is my own interpretation of this process: other authors will present you with their own variations. I have used this process as the basic structure for Part One of this book, where these stages are discussed.

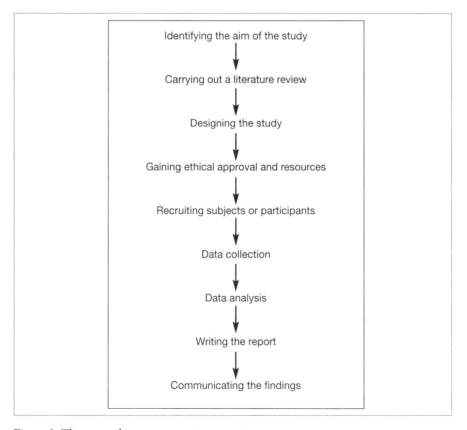

Identifying the aim of the study

↓

Carrying out a literature review

↓

Designing the study

↓

Gaining ethical approval and resources

↓

Recruiting subjects or participants

↓

Data collection

↓

Data analysis

↓

Writing the report

↓

Communicating the findings

**Figure 1** The research process – an interpretation

## EVIDENCE-BASED PRACTICE

'Evidence-based practice' also needs defining. Many health and social care professionals use the term to mean practice which is supported by research findings, but this seems to me to be rather too narrow a view. 'Evidence' includes more than just the findings of formal research projects, while simply accepting the results of a research study and applying them to every care situation is not an appropriate use of evidence.

There are many definitions of evidence-based practice, or evidence-based medicine, or evidence-based care, or whichever term might be used. One of the best known is proposed by Sackett *et al* (1997, p.2), who state that evidence-based practice is 'The conscientious, explicit and judicious use of current best evidence about the care of individual patients'.

To paraphrase, it involves using the best evidence you have about the most effective care of individuals, using it with the person's best interests in mind, to the best of your ability and in such a way that it is clear to others that you are doing it. Sackett *et al* were specifically discussing medicine, but their definition seems to apply equally well to nursing, social work, midwifery or any other related activity.

It is also important to note that Sackett *et al* refer to 'current best evidence', not to 'research evidence'. When we deliver health or social care we do not always have relevant or applicable research findings available to us. In many situations we do not have the time to look for research findings, while for other situations research has yet to be carried out. There may be other situations where research findings are available, but they are not the 'best evidence' for us.

### Key Question 2

Research findings suggest that antibiotic x is the best treatment for the ear infection that Mr Bryant is suffering from. But you know from his notes that Mr Bryant is allergic to antibiotic x. Which evidence would you use when planning Mr Bryant's care?

So if evidence can come from more than research findings, what other sources should we consider? Rycroft-Malone *et al* (2004) suggest that there are four distinct sources of evidence: research, clinical or professional experience, patients or clients and their carers, and the local context in which you practise. These sources are considered in Part Two.

I hope that you find this book interesting, enjoyable and useful. This is a tall order for any textbook, I know, and research is not always seen as the most important subject by students or practitioners in health and social care. We become health or social care practitioners in order to work with and for people, in very practical ways, and learning about the process of evidence creation seems less important than learning about doing. But health and social care practice must be driven by reliable evidence and the conscientious practitioner needs to be able to understand how this evidence is developed.

Part One

# Understanding Research

Chapter 1

# Identifying the Research Aim

This chapter discusses the first decisions in the 'research processs'.

• Why does society want health and social care research?

• Why do researchers carry out research?

• What is studied?

• What do we want to find out about it?

• The impact of these early decisions on the rest of the process.

## INTRODUCTION

Every research project has an aim. A well-written research proposal will make this aim clear to potential sponsors or supervisors of the project: a well-written research paper or report will make the aim clear to readers and potential users of the study's findings. But this overt, openly-declared, aim may not be the only one.

In this chapter we will consider the development of research aims in three forms.

1  We will consider the aim of health and social care research as a whole. We will think about why health and social care research is carried out at all, why it is seen as important for practice and worth spending so much money on every year.
2  We will think about the aim of research on a smaller scale. Why do individual academics or professionals undertake research projects or, in some cases, devote their entire careers to research?
3  We will discuss the types of aim that apply to individual research projects. We will consider both the stated, explicit, aim and the unstated, hidden, aims. We will analyse the impact that unstated aims can have on research design and consider how important it is to take them into account when we evaluate a research report.

## WHY DOES SOCIETY WANT HEALTH AND SOCIAL CARE RESEARCH?

From what I can remember, I was taught nothing about research when I was a student nurse. I have no recollection of lectures on reading research papers, understanding statistics, or critiquing research designs. My tutors, nurses and doctors alike, made few if any references to research findings during classes and my written assignments were not constrained by the need to include long lists of research papers. During practical classes and placements I was taught the 'right' way to perform a procedure, set up a dressings trolley or administer medications. No-one ever explained why this was the 'right' way, except perhaps by referring to 'experience' or 'custom and practice'.

I don't remember questioning my tutors, even when this approach to my education and to health care produced rather ridiculous practices, such as those in Key Cases 1 and 2.

### KEY CASE 1 – Injection technique

I undertook practice placements in a series of health care settings, including two major general hospitals. They have both been demolished. Last time I looked one was a car park and the other a supermarket.

In Hospital 1 intramuscular injections were given in the patient's thigh. In Hospital 2 intramuscular injections had to be given in the patient's buttock. If I was in Hospital 1 and had given an injection into a patient's buttock I would have been severely told off. If I was in Hospital 2 and had given an injection into a patient's thigh I would also have been severely told off.

## KEY CASE 2 – Hernia repairs

In Hospital 1, I worked on a male surgical ward. Many of the patients had their inguinal hernias repaired. One of the consultant surgeons insisted that every one of his patients must wear a surgical support for five days after surgery. The other consultant surgeon insisted that his patients must *not* wear surgical supports under any circumstances. Much of my time as a nurse on that ward was spent ensuring that I hadn't inadvertently given a surgical support to one of Surgeon 2's patients, or checking that all of Surgeon 1's patients were wearing their surgical supports whether they wanted to or not. Much of the rest of my time was spent trying to explain to the patients why some of them had to wear supports and some of them were not allowed to wear supports.

As a staff nurse I was never called on to back up my actions with reference to research evidence and my early years as a clinical teacher were also almost totally research free. This is not to say that no health and social care research was being done. The Royal College of Nursing had commissioned some major research projects in the mid-1970s, for example. But it rarely seemed to have any impact on my work in a series of provincial hospitals. The amount of health and social care research being undertaken started to expand more rapidly in the 1980s and 1990s, but as late as 1998 Margaret Ogier remained pessimistic about its impact on nursing: '… it is doubtful that research findings are being widely used to inform everyday practice …' (Ogier, 1998, p.5).

More recently, health and social care's adoption of an 'evidence-based' approach to practice has meant that an understanding and use of research have become more crucial for practitioners. Whether you are already qualified, or still studying to become a health or social care practitioner, you need to develop some skills in the reading and critiquing of research evidence. Much of my teaching for undergraduate and pre-registration students is about research or makes use of research findings. Student assignments are expected to refer to research and other evidence. Practice assessment requires students not only to perform skilfully but also to support their actions by referring to evidence. Gomm and Davies (2000), writing only two years after Ogier, emphasised that 'Government policy and professional guidance insist that professional practice should be "evidence-based"'.

Research is not the only source of evidence, as we have discussed, but it is an extremely influential one. Governments, international organisations, professional bodies, charities and individual patients and clients expect care to be evidence-based and expect much of the evidence to come from research. The reasons behind this move from an acceptance of custom and practice towards a demand for research evidence are complex and a discussion of them is outside the scope of this book, but the following are a few of what I think are the most important reasons.

- The public no longer trusts health and social care professionals to do what is best.
- Professionals are conscious of the risk of being sued and want clear evidence for their practices.
- Emerging health and social care professions want to create their own evidence for their roles.
- Governments demand clear evidence before funding expensive new treatments or care strategies.

So, if we want to claim that health and social care research in all its many shapes and forms has a single over-arching aim it is this: health and social care research aims to create evidence. However, while there is undoubtedly some truth to this idea, it is too simplistic to be of any real use in understanding individual projects. We also need to consider the aims of those who do research, those who pay for it and those who seek to apply it to practice. We will consider these over the next few chapters.

## WHY DO RESEARCHERS DO RESEARCH?

If society demands health and social care research, then society needs people to carry it out. These people are 'researchers', but it is a mistake to think of researchers as a single group of people, with similar backgrounds, skills and intentions. People do research, become researchers, for many different reasons.

### Key Question 1

When you hear the term 'researcher', what sort of images do you think of?

- Is a researcher someone working in a laboratory?
- Does your image incorporate test tubes, white coats and Bunsen burners?
- Or does your image contain pictures of people being interviewed, or observed going about their day-to-day lives?

Do you see yourself as a researcher?

## Who does research?

Health and social care research is done by people from many different backgrounds. Social scientists, statisticians, behavioural scientists, historians, health professionals and social care professionals all regularly undertake health and social care research. Some will be career researchers, devoting their entire working lives to researching various aspects of health and social care. At the other extreme, many health and social care professionals will undertake a small-scale research project or two while they are students and will never again take part in research.

The most typical health and social care researcher probably sits somewhere in the middle of these two extremes, combining research with practice and/or teaching. In my case, I spend about half my time teaching and half in research. Other researchers may work mostly in practice, doing occasional research projects and some teaching. We also have many different reasons for doing research.

Researchers like to think that they work to make the world a better place. Without wishing to sound too cynical, making the world a better place is more likely to be a desirable but not necessarily inevitable outcome of research rather than the primary reason for it being undertaken in the first place. Other, more mundane and less altruistic, reasons are often the primary motives behind an individual's decision to undertake a research project.

We do research because:

- we're fascinated by the cardiovascular system, or by viruses, or by the reasons why people take drugs or become criminals;
- we have a theory about the link between eating fruit and the ability to play chess and we want to test it out;
- our contracts end in a few months and we need to get a research grant so that we can extend our contracts for another year or two;
- our contracts require us to publish at least two research papers each year;
- we want to develop our reputations in our chosen fields of health or social care;
- and because we want to make the world a better place... .

## Does the reason matter?

When you are a practising health or social care professional, you will need high-quality, reliable, evidence. So does it matter why the research was carried out, providing that the findings are useful? I suggest that it does, because different reasons for doing research have an impact on what is studied, why it's studied and how it's studied. The availability of research is linked directly to the reasons why research is done.

In a perfect world, we would know everything. In an almost perfect world researchers would study those subjects that would be of most benefit to the well-being of individuals and the wider society, they would be able to fund all the necessary research and they would have the skills and resources to carry out their research effectively. In a less than perfect world, like this one, other issues arise:

- researchers' personal interests do not always correspond with the issues of most potential benefit;
- researchers don't always have the skills to undertake research in the way they would wish;
- funding organisations have their own agendas and may not wish to fund research in certain subjects, however important others might believe them to be;
- questions of interest in health and social care can be extremely complex and we do not yet have a sufficiently effective range of research methodologies and methods to answer them all.

I'm certain that many researchers strive to undertake projects that have the maximum potential benefit for patients or clients, but once real-world issues are taken into account few researchers actually develop personal research activities that achieve this aim.

## WHAT WILL BE STUDIED?

Just as there are many reasons for doing research, there are many reasons for why some subjects are heavily researched and some, apparently of equal importance, receive little attention. Decisions about what aspects of health and social care will be studied are particularly affected by issues such as:

- changing public, political or professional ideas about subjects of importance;
- emerging threats to current health and social care provision;
- new sources of research funding that are available for research into specific topics;
- new roles for health and social care professionals.

### Changing ideas

In the mid-1980s British health professionals, politicians and members of the public viewed Acquired Immune Deficiency Syndrome and Human Immunodeficiency Virus (AIDS/HIV) as a major threat to health. Its apparently sudden appearance in Western societies and its devastating effect on health meant that many people saw it as the single biggest threat to health we had to face. Research projects developed across the world, including many in the UK, and the British government allocated large sums of money to funding research. By the mid-1990s AIDS/HIV was no longer viewed with such alarm by the British public, rightly or wrongly. It was far less politically important as a result and even though it remained a major threat to health at a worldwide level, research into AIDS/HIV fell sharply.

## Emerging threats

New threats have appeared, overtaking AIDS/HIV in the minds of the public. In the mid-2000s we have seen the emergence of major public concern about nutrition and obesity, about predicted increases in the number of older people needing nursing and social care, about the emergence of Methycillin Resistant Staphylococcus Aureus (MRSA). These new threats to our social and personal well-being have created new researchers and research teams as the government and other agencies have allocated money for their study.

## New sources of funding

Changing ideas and new threats can alter the way in which research funds are allocated. Occasionally a new, rather than re-allocated, source of research funds appears and creates a shift in the ways in which money is awarded and in the subjects that are seen as appropriate for research.

The emergence of the National Lottery is a good example of a major new source of funding for research. Money from the Lottery is awarded through bodies such as the Big Lottery Fund (BLF) and much of this money is used to fund research into health and social care. Since its inception in 1995 the BLF has awarded thousands of grants. The awards include a specific funding programme for health and social care research, which gave a total of £23,623,032 to 139 projects in 1999 (Big Lottery Fund, 2007).

## New roles

The creation of new, or substantially different, roles and responsibilities for health and social care professionals also creates new research priorities and opportunities. In the past decade health care has seen the development and expansion of nurse practitioner or nurse consultant roles and the development of paramedics. Social care has seen similar developments as new ways of managing and delivering social care have impacted on the ways in which social care practitioners work.

## WHO MAKES THE DECISIONS?

At an individual level, researchers have professional and academic backgrounds, personal experiences and skills, and preferences for particular **paradigms** or **methodologies**. As a result, each researcher will tend to focus on specific subjects, issues or questions and will tend to approach them in a rather limited range of ways. I know few, if any, researchers who are equally comfortable carrying out **randomised controlled trials** of drugs and **phenomenological** studies of people's experiences of residential home care, for example.

Also, researchers in academic institutions are affected by the research aims of that institution. Most university departments will hope to develop reputations in particular fields and will actively encourage their staff to research in those fields. A department of social work may decide to focus on the study of children and families rather than the study of older people, or a medical school might decide to study infectious disease or public health rather than malignant disease or congenital problems.

## WHAT DO WE WANT TO FIND OUT?

What, in other words, will be the aim of a research project? At an informal level we often talk about research projects 'looking into' or 'studying' something, 'proving' or 'disproving' a theory or 'predicting' an effect. More formally, the aims of a research study can be classified in three ways: exploration, explanation and testing.

### Exploration

Exploratory research aims to find out about new or poorly understood phenomena. It is often viewed as an ideal 'first step' method of research, enabling the researcher to study a new, or newly altered, phenomenon when there is little, if anything, known about the subject (Thomson, 1998). This level of research can be undertaken without needing to identify complex research questions. Its research question may be no more sophisticated than asking 'What's going on here?' but this is an essential question in the early stages of investigation. Exploratory research aims to find out what's going on so that later research projects can ask more complex questions.

### KEY CASE 3 – Exploratory research projects

- *Wilson* et al *(2007)* This exploratory study focused on the experiences of foster fathers, a subject which the team found to be under-researched. The researchers used a postal questionnaire and gained responses from 69 foster fathers registered with an independent fostering agency.

- *Margetts* et al *(2006)* This project explored the experiences of grandparents of children with autistic spectrum disorders. The researchers judged that this was also an under-researched area. In contrast to Wilson *et al*, this team undertook a small-scale interview-based study of six grandparents.

## Explanation

Explanatory research seeks to arrive at a reason for the phenomenon being studied. It may follow on from the exploratory work, going on from asking 'What is happening?' to asking 'Why is this happening?' These projects may describe features of sample groups, identify **correlations** or suggest **causal relationships** (Thomson, 1998). These are important relationships to uncover, as they indicate potentially significant relationships between variables. Correlation is a measure of the link between two variables. If both variables change in the same direction (for example, both get larger, or both get faster) they are said to be positively correlated. If the variables change in opposite directions they are said to be negatively correlated. For example, if a population's life expectancy increases as it get wealthier then life expectancy and wealth are positively correlated. A causal relationship means that one variable directly causes a change in the other. Ultimately, explanatory research may generate theories.

## KEY CASE 4 – Explanatory research projects

- *Whitaker and Hirst (2002)* This explanatory project looked at the correlation between variables in the context of people with challenging behaviours. Whitaker and Hirst used a case report of a single client, showing the correlation between his outbursts of aggression and his trips outside his residential unit. The case report shows a negative correlation: in other words, as the number of trips outside grew, the number of aggressive outbursts decreased. However, the researchers emphasise that this correlation does not prove a cause-and-effect relationship: both variables might be the result of other factors.
- *Kouvonen and Lintonen (2002)* This Finnish research project studied the causal relationship between part-time working and heavy drinking among adolescents. The researchers had access to a national database and were able to analyse questionnaire responses from a total of 47,568 teenagers. The study found a significant correlation between alcohol intake and part-time work but did not find a strong causal relationship between the two variables.

## Testing

Once produced, theories need to be tested and this is the aim of the third level of research. Theories that have been successfully tested, in other words, theories that withstood rigorous testing, can be viewed as offering us widely applicable evidence about the nature of things. In health and social care such evidence should enable us to develop effective practice in a range of settings. On the other hand, theories that have been tested and disproved do not offer health and social care practitioners a basis upon which to make decisions. Research at the level of testing needs to develop its aim in such a way that it clearly defines the idea or theory that it wishes to test. This level of research, therefore, makes use of the **hypothesis**.

A hypothesis can be defined as 'a way of proposing a relationship between two or more variables, or factors' (Clifford, 1997, p.92). Wharrad (1998, p.4) describes it as a 'testable proposition about the outcome of an experiment' or an 'educated guess'. In a correlational study the researchers might simply propose that a relationship exists: for example, the hypothesis might be that there is a relationship between household income and the academic qualifications of the oldest household member. This hypothesis proposes a relationship but makes no attempt to quantify it or to establish its exact nature. In a cause-and-effect hypothesis the researcher will create a more specific hypothesis about the nature of the relationship, with one variable having a direct effect on the other. An example of this would be a hypothesis that stated that academic qualifications at PhD level will result in a higher than average household income.

Studies that set out to test hypotheses often rewrite them in a form known as the **null hypothesis**. A null hypothesis predicts no effect, or a negative relationship. So our example hypotheses would become 'there is no relationship between household income and the academic qualifications of the oldest household member' or 'academic qualifications at PhD level will not result in a higher than average household income'. Studies are then set up to test the null hypothesis and a positive result will arise when the null hypothesis is disproved. This approach is standard throughout much positivist research: studies set out to reject the idea that there is no difference, rather than prove that there is a difference. Many studies will seek to test more than one hypothesis, leading to extremely complex reports on multiple measurements and outcomes.

### KEY CASE 5 – Research testing hypotheses

- *Parry and Lindsay (2003)* The researchers set out to test the hypothesis that sexual offenders who have intellectual disabilities would have higher impulsiveness scores than people with intellectual disabilities who were not sexual offenders. Forty-one men were recruited to the study: 22 who had committed sexual offences and 19 who had not. The impulsiveness scores of each participant were recorded and analysed. The results suggested that the sexual offenders were actually less impulsive than the other participants, thus disproving the hypothesis. You should note that unlike many hypothesis-testing studies this project did not present a null hypothesis, nor did it use an experimental design. This is a good example of a project that does not conform to the very narrow view of research held by some practitioners: it draws on different methodologies and methods to put together a study which the researchers believe will be the best way of achieving their aim.

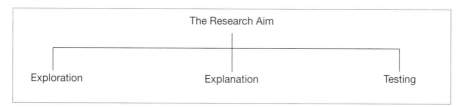

**Figure 1** A classification of research aims

## ACHIEVING SUCCESS

Ultimately, the success of a research project can be measured only on its completion. But before a research project begins we need to be able to predict the likelihood of success. The aim, therefore, cannot be established in isolation. The researcher has also to have some idea of the resources that are likely to be available, the chance of achieving funding, the likelihood of being able to recruit enough participants or subjects, the methods of data collection and analysis that are to be employed.

I might decide to carry out a research project with the aim of discovering a cure for all known infectious diseases. Most people would agree that this is a worthy aim, but few people would consider it to be a realistic one. Even if I was a leading expert on infectious disease I doubt that I would be taken seriously. The history of health and social care is not a history of sudden giant leaps and earth-shattering achievements, it's a history of small steps, of minor improvements that add together over time to create major change. For every great leap forward there are hundreds or even thousands of tiny changes.

On the other hand, some changes might be too tiny to be worth bothering about. If curing all known infectious diseases is rather too ambitious, I could set up an observational study to establish how many people attending a social services day centre on a particular Tuesday afternoon arrive wearing blue hats. It's a low-risk project, as well as low cost. I can probably collect accurate data, provided that I define 'blue' and 'hat' sufficiently clearly. But what's the aim? A research project is not necessarily worthwhile just because it's *achievable*: it must also be potentially *useful*. In other words, the aim of a research project should be grounded in an understanding of what might be achievable: the researcher needs to understand the conditions under which the research will take place. As a reader of research papers you, too, need to understand these conditions in order to be able to judge the project's success.

In the following chapters we will consider in detail many of the factors that influence individual research projects and affect their aims and the likelihood that they will achieve them.

---

## KEY LEARNING POINTS

- Health and social care has moved from a foundation in custom, practice and experience to a focus on evidence-based care delivery.
- Research is a central activity in the creation of this evidence base.
- Individual researchers undertake projects with a variety of aims in mind, not only the advancement of health and social care.
- Research project aims may be exploration, explanation or the testing of ideas.
- A project's aim must be realistic, achievable and potentially *useful*.

---

## FURTHER READING

Brechin, A and Sidell, M (2000) 'Ways of knowing', in Gomm, R and Davies, C (eds) *Using evidence in health and social care*. London: Open University/Sage

Clifford, C (1997) *Nursing and health care research* (2nd edn). London: Prentice Hall

Krauss, SE (2005) 'Research paradigms and meaning making: a primer'. *The Qualitative Report*, 10: 758–70

Lanoe, N (2002) *Ogier's reading Research* (3rd edn). London: Baillière Tindall

Thomson, AM (1998) 'Recognizing research processes in research-based literature', in Crookes, PA and Davies, S (eds) *Research into practice*. Edinburgh: Baillière Tindall

**Chapter 2**

# Reviewing the Literature

This chapter discusses how to evaluate existing research evidence.

- Developing a search strategy.

- Searching the databases.

- Evaluating quality.

## INTRODUCTION

In almost every health and social care research project, a literature review will be carried out at an early stage and its results will influence the researcher's decisions about project design. Literature reviews occur at every level of research, whether the intended project is large-scale and multi-national or small-scale and local. They are frequently the first structured and organised investigations undertaken by health and social care professionals. Many of you might be reading this book in preparation for a literature review of your own. A particular, specialist, form of literature review, the **systematic review**, is one of the most important sources of evidence for health and social care practice and a form of research in its own right. A well-planned and efficiently undertaken literature review can be a far more useful piece of work than a small-scale primary research project. But many literature reviews are poorly designed and badly executed, leading to **biased** and unreliable results.

In this chapter we will consider the key qualities of an effective literature review and discuss the different activities needed to achieve one. Because many of you will need to review literature yourselves, I will try to provide some hints and tips to make the activity easier for you.

## WHY DOES A RESEARCHER NEED TO KNOW WHAT'S ALREADY AVAILABLE?

When I plan a research project I have three aims in carrying out a review of the literature. I want:

1  to understand the context in which my project will take place;
2  to understand the evidence provided by existing research;
3  to establish if my intended project can be justified.

If you are about to carry out a literature review as a way of informing your health or social care practice, then the first two points still apply. However, I think you should replace the third aim with another one:

• to decide whether or not the evidence I find can be appropriately applied to practice.

We will discuss this last aim in Chapter 8. At this point I want us to concentrate on the first three aims.

## UNDERSTANDING THE CONTEXT

• How much research is already out there?
• Where does it come from?
• Who has produced it?
• Who paid for it?
• What methods have been used to produce it?
• How old is it?

These are some of the most important questions about the context of my proposed new project. They are also questions that can usefully be applied to the entire spectrum of health and social care research and, thankfully, they are usually easy to answer.

### How much research already exists?

A good search strategy should help us to establish how much research already exists. It is not yet possible to identify every single research publication that may be relevant, but it is possible to find increasingly greater proportions of the literature.

In some cases thousands, even tens of thousands, of publications might be available. Other subjects may have far fewer research papers available, particularly if they are recent problems or are not considered to be of major importance to health or social services. Another important factor to consider is the fact that each database will list different collections of papers.

## KEY CASE 1 – Examples of search results

I searched three databases, using simple keyword searches: 'child protection', 'child abuse' and 'cancer'. In each database I searched for the 25-year period 1982–2007.

For 'child protection':

- Cumulative Index to Nursing and Allied Health Literature (CINAHL) (1982–2007) – 575 results;
- International Bibliography of the Social Sciences (IBSS) (1982–2007) – 373 results;
- MEDLINE (1982–2007) – 553 results.

For 'Child abuse':

- CINAHL (1982–2007) – 6,978 results;
- IBSS (1982–2007) – 425 results;
- MEDLINE (1982–2007) – 15,806 results.

For 'cancer':

- CINAHL (1982–2007) – 48,008 results;
- IBSS (1982–2007) – 1,009 results;
- MEDLINE (1982–2007) – 478,756 results.

Before I undertook these searches I felt fairly confident that IBSS would return the greatest number of references (or 'hits') for both 'child protection' and 'child abuse' as these terms refer to a problem which routinely involves social care professionals. This did not turn out to be the case and IBSS produced fewer hits than either CINAHL or MEDLINE. I expected MEDLINE to return the largest number of hits using 'cancer' as the search term, but I was surprised at the number of references it identified. MEDLINE returned ten times as many references as CINAHL and over 450 times more than IBSS.

I could of course have limited my search in many different ways, some of which we will discuss later in this chapter. Doing so would have resulted in far fewer hits and would have made it much easier for me to consider each of the references individually. But these quick searches do clearly show that the choice of database can produce markedly different results. If you want to undertake a comprehensive search for evidence, leading to a genuine understanding of the quantity of material that is available, then you should always search more than one database.

## Where is it from?

Is the research from the UK, the USA, China or South Africa? Is it from hospital or community settings? Urban or rural environments? Does the location of the project affect its relevance to my proposed study? If you are interested in the effects of a drug on a disease then the location of the study may not be critical. Indeed, drug trials are intended to be generalisable, so the results of a study in London should be generalisable to the same situation in New York or Beijing. But if you are interested in finding out about how to reduce wrist injuries in cricket players, will a study of wrist injury prevention in American baseball players be useful, or will a study of wrist injuries in catering staff in Stockholm be of value? Possibly, but their applicability might be less obvious.

## Who did it?

Researchers are influenced by their professional and academic backgrounds, so establishing these backgrounds can be useful. If psychiatrists study depression, for example, their research questions and methodologies are likely to differ from the questions and methodologies that would be found in projects undertaken by social workers or mental health nurses. A multi-professional team might produce a more balanced approach to research.

It is not always easy to identify the qualifications or professional or academic backgrounds of researchers. Many journals list author qualifications and job titles but others do not and may identify nothing more than an author's place of work. A researcher from a 'Faculty of Health and Social Care' could be a physician, physiotherapist, psychologist or statistician. If you feel, as a reader, that knowing more about a researcher is critical then you will need to investigate further.

## Who paid?

If a research project was funded this is usually indicated by an acknowledgement in each publication that arises from the project. The amount of funding is never revealed, but the source of the funding is shown. You might feel that funding by certain organisations might lead to bias, or undue pressure to come up with particular results. This is unlikely to be the case nowadays, but a study of the effects of smoking paid for by a tobacco company or a study of stress in a workforce paid for by the workers' trade union might be open to accusations of bias, however ill-founded they might be.

## What methods?

Is the available research from a single **paradigm**, using a narrow range of methodologies and data? Or does it reflect a more varied approach, with a mix of project designs and methods of data collection and analysis? If a subject has been studied many times using a narrow range of methods then a new project using a design from a different paradigm may produce original and worthwhile insights. Or perhaps existing studies have always investigated the same population. Focusing on a different group, children instead of adults for example, might prove instructive.

## How old is the current literature?

There may be plenty of research available, but perhaps only from the last four or five years. Or there may be plenty of papers written in the early 1980s and the mid-1990s but none from the last ten years. Health and social care practice changes rapidly and research may go out of date in only a year or two. So older research papers may no longer be relevant however well-designed the studies were. On the other hand, there are many classic or seminal research papers that are still relevant even many years after they were published, such as the work of John Bowlby or Jean Piaget in the field of child development.

## UNDERSTANDING THE EXISTING EVIDENCE

The first set of questions (page 14) is a valuable one and can help you to understand a great deal about the origins and nature of existing evidence. But these questions don't enable you to understand the *conclusions* reached by this research or the *quality* of individual research papers. Achieving an understanding of what the existing evidence claims and how well it supports its claims is a more difficult part of the literature review.

The contextual questions regarding the funding of a project or the qualifications of a researcher can often be answered simply by reading the title of a research paper and its abstract. To understand the conclusions of a paper and to judge its quality you need to explore the paper in much more detail. You need to read the paper, unsurprisingly, but your reading can be helped by the use of a framework or model. There are many such models or frameworks available and I will refer to them collectively as appraisal tools. We will be looking at some examples shortly.

I'd like to add a note of caution here. Many literature reviews, whether written by students, experienced practitioners or even lecturers, seem to make the assumption that because a research paper has been published that means the research project was of good quality. The writers end up reporting the findings of projects without questioning the research that produced them. This can be dangerous.

- Published research is not automatically good-quality research.
- Qualifications do not make you an expert.

Remembering these two statements should help you to avoid being too accepting of research reports. Literature reviews should always be produced critically. To do so you need an understanding of research and a consistent approach to appraisal.

## CAN I JUSTIFY MY PROJECT?

Achieving the first two aims, understanding the research context and evaluating the conclusions and quality of existing evidence, enables you to judge if your own study can be justified. If you feel that you can justify the development of your project then you can move on to the next stage. If you feel unable to justify your project then you will need to think again. Figure 1 gives you some of the conclusions a researcher might reach.

| Probably | Probably not |
|---|---|
| There is no existing research.<br><br>Existing research is no longer relevant because the situation has changed.<br><br>Existing research is poor quality.<br><br>No-one has studied the subject in the way I want to. | There are many high-quality studies already.<br><br>There is little existing research but it all reaches the same conclusion.<br><br>My proposed study is almost identical to an earlier one. |

**Figure 1** Can I justify my study?

## CARRYING OUT THE LITERATURE REVIEW

The good news is that the internet has made access to research papers far easier than it has ever been. The bad news is that an effective literature review still needs to be planned and carried out in an organised way. Indeed, the internet offers so many potential resources that the task of carrying out a literature review might actually be more complex and complicated than it used to be. There are four stages to a successful literature review:

1 developing a search strategy;
2 searching the databases;
3 retrieving relevant papers;
4 evaluating their quality.

## DEVELOPING A SEARCH STRATEGY

To develop an effective strategy a researcher needs to answer two questions:

1 What am I looking for?
2 Where am I likely to find it?

### What am I looking for?

A review needs to have clear criteria for what literature to consider. The inclusion criteria define what makes a paper suitable for the review, while exclusion criteria establish what makes a paper unsuitable. Exclusion criteria are not merely the opposite of inclusion criteria. They set out characteristics that make a paper irrelevant even if it meets the inclusion criteria.

Inclusion and exclusion criteria are also useful when it comes to recruiting subjects or participants for a study and will be discussed in relation to recruitment in Chapter 5.

Initially, researchers may set quite narrow inclusion criteria for the review, particularly if the subject has been heavily researched. For example:

- papers published no more than five years ago;
- papers published in English;
- **randomised controlled trials**;
- research conducted in the UK or Europe.

If these criteria produce insufficient material for the review then they can be revised, to include older studies or work from more countries perhaps.

## Where am I likely to find it?

The internet offers many databases. A database is basically a vast electronic store of information, with the major benefit that it can be searched by using a series of words or phrases in order to provide the researcher with a list of publications that may be of interest. Most of the leading databases enable the researcher to link directly to a copy of an article, if available. The leading health and social care databases include:

- MEDLINE;
- CINAHL;
- ASSIA;
- IBSS;
- Embase;
- Pubmed.

All health and social care research databases do the same basic job. You enter your search terms into the database's search box, click a button and wait a few seconds for the database to provide you with a list of relevant references.

Simple, isn't it.

But searching for literature is not the simple, foolproof, process that researchers often make it out to be. Students often tell me that it is one of the most frustrating activities they have to undertake. There are two main reasons for this: no two databases operate in exactly the same way or list exactly the same selection of references, and no two researchers use exactly the same words or phrases to describe things such as research methods or approaches to care.

## SEARCHING THE DATABASES

You know the subject you are interested in. This in turn should enable you to draw up a list of possible sources of information. If your subject is most closely related to health care then MEDLINE or Pubmed is likely to be of use. If there is a strong nursing focus then CINAHL might be a good starting-point. Social care subjects are most likely to appear in ASSIA. Increasingly, students and researchers alike start with a search in Google Scholar, a free database that enables you to carry out a wide-ranging search across academic disciplines or to narrow your search within certain related groups of disciplines.

Because databases don't overlap exactly, most researchers will need to search more than one. Some services enable more than one database to be searched at the same time: Ovid, for example, allows up to seven different databases to be searched simultaneously using the same search terms. Other databases, such as Google Scholar or the Campbell Collaboration or Cochrane Libraries, have to be searched individually.

## Using search terms

The key to a successful database search is the use of accurate search terms and a consistent approach to setting your search parameters. Knowing how to use search terms and parameters is as important as knowing which databases to search. Choosing the right ones can save valuable time and effort. A discussion of all the possible terms and parameters is outside the scope of this book, but you might find the following to be useful.

- *Truncation* – using a special symbol to shorten a search term in order to search for all the different endings of the term. In Key Case 2 (see page 23), for example, using 'epilep$' will ensure that 'epilepsy', 'epilepsies' and 'epileptic' are all searched for.
- *Boolean operators* – these are terms such as 'AND', 'OR' or 'NOT'. They enable you to combine searches containing keywords of interest, or to exclude hits that contain unwanted terms. For example, 'community AND care' would search for references including both terms, 'community OR care' would search for references containing either term and 'community NOT care' would search for references that contained the first term but not the second. The AND search would include references to 'community care' and also references in which the terms appeared separately.
- *Language* – if you are not able to understand more than one language then you can limit your search to papers in that language. I expect that most of you would wish to limit your searches to English language references: in the databases I refer to this will usually exclude only a small number of references.
- *Date of publication* – there is no need to search for references from every available year unless you are undertaking a **systematic review**. At first, try limiting your search to the most recent five years. If this is insufficient you can always expand the search later.
- *Other strategies* – these are too numerous to mention in detail, but Key Case 2 (page 23) offers one or two more examples. 'EXP', short for 'explode', makes the database search for the indicated term and all those related to it. 'ADJ' enables you to search for words that are adjacent to each other.

## Key Question 1: Exploring research databases

Choose two databases which enable you to search for health or social care research papers. Choose a simple single-word search term: 'homeless', perhaps, or 'bronchitis'.

For each database enter your chosen term into the search box. How many references does each database find? How many references occur in both databases and how many are found by one database only?

Now apply some limits to your search. The available limits will depend on the databases you have chosen but will usually include things like year of publication or language. How does each limiting factor affect the results? Do the limits make your search more useful or less useful?

## Sensitivity and specificity

A successful literature search will ensure that you find as many relevant sources of information as possible. One way of doing this is to undertake the search in two stages.

- Stage 1 aims for sensitivity and uses a search strategy.
- Stage 2 aims for specificity and requires the appraisal of individual references.

In Stage 1 a sensitive search is undertaken to find as many potentially relevant references as possible. Search terms are combined in such a way as to ensure that they cover all possible terms, spellings and descriptions of sources. As a result, this stage of the search should produce a long list of references. Within this list there should be a high proportion of your required sources, which is the positive outcome of a sensitive search. The negative outcome is that the search will also have presented you with a large number of ultimately irrelevant references.

Stage 2 will separate the relevant references from the irrelevant ones. This stage involves a more detailed appraisal of each reference to ensure that it meets the inclusion criteria for the search but does not also match any of the exclusion criteria. The researcher will need to check each reference in turn, discarding those that do not meet the inclusion criteria. In some cases a quick look at the title of the reference will be sufficient, in other cases the abstract will need to be read. Occasionally neither of these will be sufficient and the researcher will need to access the full version of the paper before reaching a decision.

In very detailed literature searchs such as those needed in systematic reviews a very high proportion of the papers identified in Stage 1 will be rejected: often well over 95%. The fact that so many papers from Stage 1 are rejected at Stage 2 might surprise you and suggest that Stage 1 is very inefficient, but this is not the case. Stage 1 must use broad inclusion criteria because databases and article titles are not that efficient at providing accurate information. Journal editors now expect article titles to be more informative than in the past, with each title ideally giving a hint of the subject of the study, the methods used and the population targeted, but this has been the case in only the last few years. Older articles often have strange and uninformative titles that offer few hints of their content. Similarly, databases can be inaccurate or can miscategorise papers, so that a paper listed as being based on a randomised trial turns out to be a case study, or a paper identified as relating to adolescents studied only adults. Stage 2 ensures that these problems are overcome by the reviewers.

---

**KEY CASE 2 – Search strategy for a Cochrane review (from Bradley and Lindsay, 2007)**

 1  exp EPILEPSY/
 2  epilep$.mp.
 3  1 or 2
 4  exp Ambulatory Care/
 5  exp Health Care Delivery/
 6  exp Program Evaluation/
 7  exp 'Outcomes (Health Care)'/
 8  (centre$ or center$).mp.
 9  nurs$.mp.
10  specialist$.mp.
11  (epilep$ adj4 (centre$ or center$)).mp.
12  (epilep$ adj3 nurs$).mp.
13  (epilep$ adj3 specialist$).mp.
14  4 or 5 or 6 or 7
15  3 and 14
16  11 or 12 or 13 or 15

---

## WHAT ELSE SHOULD BE SEARCHED?

For any subject in health and social care my first means of obtaining information is always to access internet databases. But for a truly comprehensive search for information I will always use other sources of information as well. As I have already said, the internet is still not the source of all knowledge: older sources of information are still of value.

## The library

Many researchers and students still prefer to start their searches in the library. A college or university library is a vast repository of information, much of which will not be accessible electronically. Most textbooks, for example, have yet to be made available on the internet and many older journal articles are still accessible only in hard-copy form. However, health and social care practice changes frequently and is constantly being influenced by new policies or research findings, so a genuinely comprehensive literature search should include, but not be limited exclusively to, the library.

## Grey literature

Not all research projects result in a journal article or a book being published. Small-scale projects, projects undertaken to gain a qualification, projects that did not produce particularly insightful findings, or projects produced for specific organisations or funding bodies may get no further than the production of a dissertation, thesis or limited-circulation report. This material is referred to as grey literature. In a fully comprehensive literature search, such as that undertaken in the development of a systematic review, grey literature must also be searched for.

### Key Question 2: Searching for policies and guidelines

As a practitioner you need to be able to assess policy or guideline documents as well as research papers. Many such documents can be found if you search the databases, but in other cases it might be useful to go directly to an organisation's website.

Choose two organisations, one government department and one large policy-making organisation (for example, the Department for Education and Skills or the National Institute for Health and Clinical Excellence). Using the search terms you used in Key Question 1 (page 22) carry out a search on each of these websites.

- How effective was your search this time?
- Can you apply limits?
- How do these compare to the limits in the databases?

## EVALUATING QUALITY

Once the literature search is over, the researcher is left with a selection of references which meet the inclusion criteria. Before these are incorporated in the literature review there is one final stage of appraisal: evaluating the quality of the work.

Not every literature review undertakes this stage. Many reviews, carried out by experienced researchers as well as by students or junior academics, seem to pay little attention to the quality of a reference and appear happy to refer to the results of a piece of research without considering whether the project was reliable, valid or trustworthy.

If you simply want to ascertain how much research exists on a particular topic then an appraisal tool is unnecessary: you are interested in quantity not quality. However, I would recommend the use of an appraisal tool in every literature review. It will offer a useful structure on which you can base your appraisal and will help you to ensure consistency across each of the papers you critique.

## Choosing an appraisal tool

There are at least 121 published critical appraisal tools in existence (Katrak *et al*, 2004). They can be classified in two main ways.

1 General tools or specific tools. General tools are designed to appraise any research project, whatever its design may be. An example is the strategy developed by Gould (1994), which features 47 questions in 13 sections. Specific tools are intended for the appraisal of specific research designs. They include the CASP series of tools, provided by the Public Health Resource Unit (2006). There are seven appraisal tools in this series, each specific to one type of research design.
2 Tools that provide general 'checklist' style guidelines for research appraisal and those where your appraisal results in a numerical score.

Your choice of appraisal tool is likely to be based on personal preference, unless you are directed to make use of a specific tool. In a general literature review, which you undertake in order to gain an understanding of the overall quality of research, the choice of tool is probably not critical. In cases where an assessment of the quality of individual papers is vital then the choice of appraisal tool is more important. What I find particularly interesting about critical appraisal tools is that most of them have not been developed using empirical approaches and have not been tested in use, so they are not of proven **validity** or **reliability**. Indeed, Katrak *et al* found that only 14 appraisal tools (12%) had been developed in a systematic, evidence-based fashion. A lack of consistency in the development of appraisal tools means that the same research report can be given markedly different quality assessments depending on which tools are used to appraise it.

## SUMMARY

Health and social care practitioners must be able to identify and evaluate literature if they are to understand their practice fully. Searching for literature should not be a haphazard activity: it needs a logical and consistent approach and the more you practise literature searching the easier it becomes. Once you have identified literature of interest it is important that you do not simply take it at face value and accept what it has to say. It is vital that you read the literature critically, being on the lookout for problems as well as for the vital points that may have a direct impact on your practice. Once again, there are tools and frameworks that can help you to critique literature successfully, but regular reading and critiquing will soon help you to develop your skills so that critical reading becomes almost second nature to you.

---

### KEY LEARNING POINTS

What characterises a good literature review?

- Based on a comprehensive and transparent search strategy.
- Uses clear inclusion and exclusion criteria.
- Aims for sensitivity and specificity.
- Appraises quality as well as quantity.
- Is written critically.

---

## FURTHER READING

Gould, D (1994) 'Writing literature reviews'. *Nurse Researcher*, 2: 13–23

Katrak, P, Bialocerkowski, AE, Massy-Westropp, N, Saravana Kumar, VS and Grimmer, KA (2004) 'A systematic review of the content of critical appraisal tools'. BMC *Medical Research Methodology*, 4: 22

**www.biomedcentral.com/1471-2288/4/22** (7 March 2007). This short paper evaluates critical appraisal tools. While it doesn't offer you a step-by-step method of appraisal it does include some interesting discussion about the validity of appraisal tools.

Lanoe, N (2002) *Ogier's reading research.* (3rd edn). London: Baillière Tindall

Lee, P (2006) 'Understanding some naturalistic research methodologies'. *Paediatric Nursing*, 18: 44–6

Public Health Resource Unit (2006) *Critical appraisal tools.* **www.phru.nhs.uk/casp/critical_appraisal_tools.htm** (7 March 2007). The CASP critical appraisal tools can all be found on this site. They are the tools I recommend to students. Each tool is designed for use with a specific type of research method, so you do need to know what method a study used in order to select the appropriate appraisal tool, which can be a drawback if this information is not clearly given.

# Chapter 3

# Designing a Study

This chapter discusses research design.

- Defining paradigms, methodologies, methods and tools.

- The major paradigms – positivist and interpretive.

- The major methodologies – experimental and naturalistic.

- The major methods – qualitative, quantitative, mixed.

- The 'research hierarchies'.

- External influences on research design.

## INTRODUCTION

In this chapter we will be looking at some of the key factors that influence the ways in which research projects are designed. Once a research aim or question has been finalised, decisions about these factors will lead to the design of the project.

There are many ways in which a research project can be designed. However, this is not as complicated a process as it might appear, because not all possibilities are open to every researcher or to every project. Health and social care researchers are not, in my experience, experts in all possible research methods. We are all the results of our experience, ideas and education and so we tend to have preferences and skills in some areas but not in others. Some of us are expert statisticians, some are skilled interviewers, some can develop high-quality observational studies and others can design and manage complex, multi-centre clinical trials. We all have our own combinations of skills, preferences, weaknesses and uncertainties.

The design of a research project is the result of decisions made at three main levels: about the **paradigm**, the **methodology** and the method. Each level of decision-making affects the levels beneath it, gradually creating a unique combination of choices and, ultimately, the project itself.

## THE THREE LEVELS

### Paradigms

A research paradigm is 'a general theory that informs most scholarship on the operation and outcomes of any particular system of thought and action' (Entman, 1993, p.56). In other words, it's a system of beliefs and ideas about the best way to find out about the world and, therefore, about research itself. Every health and social care researcher has a paradigm, even if they don't think consciously about what this paradigm might be. We all have ideas and beliefs about the best way to understand the world, especially health and social care, and this set of beliefs has a big influence on how we do research and what we study.

### Key Question 1 – What's your paradigm?

Think about the following questions and discuss them with colleagues or in class. If you haven't thought about these questions before you might find them hard to answer, but try to do so honestly. Remember, there is no single 'correct' paradigm.

- What do you think about the best ways to investigate the world?
- What do you think about the best ways to investigate health and social care questions?
- Do you prefer to observe things, or to get in there and make changes?

### Methodologies

These are broad approaches to the design of research projects. Methodology means, strictly speaking, 'the study of method'. However, in modern research the word is used to refer to the ways in which a project can be designed. A methodology is, therefore, the 'strategy, plan of action, process or design lying behind the choice and use of particular methods and linking the choice and use of methods to the desired outcomes' (Brechin and Sidell, 2000, p.7). Methodologies are concerned particularly with the extent to which a research project should alter or control the situation in which research takes place, how it should collect data and how this data can be analysed. Although methodologies can be divided into two basic classes, each of these classes can be subdivided into a range of distinctive and more closely defined approaches.

## Methods

The different ways in which individual research projects can carry out key functions, such as recruitment and selection, data collection and data analysis, are the research methods.

There are many different research methods although, as we will see shortly, they can also usefully be gathered under two main headings. Once the methods have been chosen this, in turn, leads to a further set of decisions about the tools to be used within the project.

## MAKING SENSE OF THE LEVELS

Your understanding of these different levels of choice might be made more difficult by the fact that the choices are not presented consistently in the literature.

When it comes to paradigms this inconsistency is especially obvious. Brechin and Sidell (2000) refer to positivist and interpretivist paradigms. Lee (2006) talks of the naturalistic paradigm. Burke Johnson and Onwuegbuzie (2004) propose three paradigms: quantitative, qualitative and mixed methods. Krauss (2005) also suggests three paradigms, but calls them qualitative or naturalistic/constructivist, quantitative or positivist, and realist.

There is more consistency regarding methodologies, with most authors referring to two types, qualitative and quantitative (for example, Krauss, 2005; Onwuegbuzie and Leech, 2005; Hart *et al*, 2005). However, Lee (2006) uses the terms naturalistic and qualitative interchangeably while Brechin and Sidell (2000, p.9) take a completely different approach and refer to the 'methodological frameworks' of 'hypothesis testing', 'addressing research questions' and 'hermeneutic enquiry'.

Methods also tend to be divided into two types, with most authors continuing with the quantitative and qualitative categories (for example, Malterud, 2001). However, Brechin and Sidell (2000) appear reluctant to use such a simple classification, choosing instead to list a range of 15 methods relating to their three methodologies.

The debate is complicated even further by the way in which terms are used and by the lack of clarity about what many of them mean to the authors who use them. Neale *et al* (2005) use qualitative and quantitative to refer to paradigms, methodologies *and* methods. Other writers use terms such as 'designs', 'approaches', 'traditions' or 'strategies' synonymously with 'methods' and 'methodologies' (for example, Concato *et al*, 2000; Shaw, 2003; Hart *et al*, 2005). Crucial debates about key concepts in the research process are undertaken without a consistent and clear under-standing of the choices that are available and the ways in which these choices can be made.

## My approach

To help in ensuring consistency and clarity in this book I have developed a classification of these key concepts based on my own views about health and social care research as well as on those expressed by other researchers. I have deliberately chosen to use different terms at each level as well. This should help you to avoid confusion between paradigms and methodologies, or between methodologies and methods. In my classification these are the terms I have chosen:

- Paradigms – Positivist or Interpretivist.
- Methodologies – Experimental or Naturalistic (and their subdivisions).
- Methods – Quantitative or Qualitative (and their subdivisions).

This is not a classification that will meet with every health and social care researcher's approval. However, it makes clear distinctions between levels, avoiding the confusion that can arise if every level is referred to by using the same terms.

## PARADIGMS

### Positivist or interpretive?

The positivist paradigm proposes that 'data and its analysis are value-free and data do not change because they are being observed' (Krauss, 2005, p.760) and that 'inquiry should be objective' (Burke Johnson and Onwuegbuzie, 2004, p.14). Positivist research focuses on 'generalisability and causal explanation' (Brechin and Sidell, 2000, p.10): on explaining **causal relationships** in such a way that these explanations can be applied to all similar relationships wherever they occur. Many people think of positivism as 'the scientific approach', establishing 'facts' through tightly controlled investigations that collect 'objective' data. You might find it helpful to think of positivism as the predictive approach to research: positivists want to create information that enables them to predict what will happen in the future. Research into the likely changes in the world's climate, or the effect of drug x on disease y, or on the link between nutrition and behaviour, is likely to be positivist.

The interpretive paradigm focuses on 'relativism and understanding' (Brechin and Sidell, 2000, p.10), hence it can also be called the relativist paradigm. Interpretive researchers 'contend that multiple-constructed realities abound …' (Burke Johnson and Onwuegbuzie, 2004, p.14) and they are not concerned with establishing relationships that can be used to predict events elsewhere. They believe that each situation, event or experience is viewed uniquely by each individual: each person experiences their own reality. By understanding these multiple realities we can come to understand more about the situation or event.

A positivist researcher might try to explain a football match by collecting and analysing data about the size of the crowd, the number of goals scored, the distance covered by each player, the number of fouls committed by each team and other numerical data. An interpretive researcher might try to understand it by interviewing fans, players and officials about their emotions during a game, by attending the match and then writing about their own feelings and by asking a selection of fans and players to keep diaries about the days leading up to the game. Of course, a researcher could combine the two paradigms and try to understand the match through using objective and subjective data, but this approach is surprisingly rare in health and social care research.

Some researchers hold very strong beliefs about which paradigm is the 'right one' and will always design projects with this in mind. For example, many medical researchers believe that the positivist paradigm is superior when we try to understand how health or social care works, so they would insist that evidence must come from experimental studies and statistical data. Other researchers, myself included, are more flexible, believing that each paradigm has strengths and weaknesses and choosing the paradigm which they feel is the most appropriate for a particular subject.

## How can you tell which paradigm has been chosen?

In some cases a research paper will identify its chosen paradigm, perhaps comparing it to alternative ones: the choice is made explicit. In other cases the paradigm will not be mentioned but you may still be able to identify it by picking up clues in the text: the choice is implicit.

Interestingly, I find that the choice of paradigm is more likely to be explicit when researchers decide to follow the interpretive paradigm and more likely to be implicit when researchers follow the positivist paradigm. I think this is probably because positivist researchers tend to feel more confident in their choice and assume that readers share their belief. Interpretive researchers often seem to be less confident and feel that they must justify their choice of paradigm in every paper.

Knowing what paradigm a researcher supports can be interesting. It helps you to understand why the research has been carried out in a particular way and can help you to understand what **bias** may affect the project. But for most health and social care professionals, who want to know if a piece of research can help their practice, such knowledge isn't vital. Understanding the methodology and the methods is far more important.

# METHODOLOGY

## Experimental or naturalistic?

Does the research set up a false, controlled, situation within which it will study its chosen subject: is it creating an experiment? Or does the project collect data from the 'real world', without altering relationships and events: is it naturalistic?

An experimental methodology can set up what amounts to an alternative reality, within which every aspect of the physical environment, interactions, behaviours and relationships can be tightly controlled. It can put rats in a maze, or it can place human beings in situations that are completely managed by the research team. Within these controlled settings, the experimenters can ensure that whatever variable they wish to study can be identified and isolated. In health and social care such total control of the environment is not always possible, but here too an experimental methodology can, through careful use of **sampling** and **randomisation**, for example, produce a controlled situation within which it can modify subjects' behaviours and produce evidence. Experimental methodologies include **randomised controlled trials** and **cohort studies**.

Such an ability would seem to be able to produce high-quality research evidence, but it is not without its problems. One of the main problems with experimental research is that it is experimental. It is setting up false situations and controls and if these situations can't be found in real life then it is unlikely that its findings will translate to real situations either. Health and social care practice takes place in the real world, not in experimental situations, and opponents of the experimental approach to gathering evidence are always quick to point this out.

Naturalistic research tries not to alter the situations it's interested in. Instead, it observes these situations either directly or indirectly, using methodologies such as **ethnography**, **grounded theory** or **phenomenology**. Ethnography is the study of a culture or community using a range of fieldwork methods including observation and interviews. In classic ethnographic studies the researchers moved into cultures very different from their own and lived in them for months or even years. In health and social care research ethnography is usually on a much smaller scale. Grounded theory is a form of research which uses careful coding and classification of data to enable theories to emerge from the information as it is analysed. A characteristic of this approach is constant comparison, where early data is analysed in order to begin the coding and classification process and in order to influence later stages of collection and analysis, unlike many methodologies where data analysis doesn't start until collection is complete.

Naturalistic studies often use small numbers of participants, discovering large amounts of information in order to create 'thick descriptions'. They can be extremely good at enabling us to understand what it means to be in a particular situation or to experience a specific event, but they are not so good at producing evidence that can be generalised to other situations in different places. Phenomenology is a good example of this. I find it to be one of the hardest research methods to understand. D.W. Smith (2003) defines it as 'the study of "phenomena": appearances of things, or things as they appear in our experience, or the ways we experience things … Phenomenology studies conscious experience as experienced from the subjective or first person point of view'. This is quite a clear definition and it focuses on phenomenology's emphasis on the 'lived experience' of individuals, which makes it very attractive to health and social care researchers. But it hides the complexity of this methodology, with its different 'subtypes' and its seemingly ever-changing approaches to the acts of data collection and analysis. That makes it hard to understand, at least for me.

At a very basic level, experimental methodologies set up experiments and naturalistic methodologies study things in their normal or natural settings. However, as with health and social care practice, health and social care research isn't that simple. Many projects take place in natural environments, but deliberately alter them in order to create an experiment. Many naturalistic projects need to alter the normal environment in order to carry out the research, although they will attempt to minimise these alterations. You can, of course, find research projects that are genuinely experimental or naturalistic, but these are in the minority in health and social care research.

An example of a pure experimental methodology would be the study of cellular-level disease processes undertaken in a laboratory. The conditions in the laboratory, the methods used, the equipment, the cells and microorganisms being studied, can all be tightly controlled. The entire study can be replicated in different laboratories across the world. Experiments such as these are carried out, for example, in the early stages of research into new drugs or vaccines and are crucial to the development of health care.

Experimental laboratory studies may be vital, but health and social care professionals are more interested in how a new drug or vaccine will work for people in their normal lives. So most of the experimental research you are likely to read about will be undertaken in situations that cannot be completely controlled.

A naturalistic study that does not alter the setting in which it takes place would need to be a secret study. You could, for example, set up hidden cameras and microphones in a residential home and study the behaviour of staff and residents. However, health and social care research needs to be ethical and a key feature of ethical research is that a person needs to give **informed consent** in order to take part. Once someone knows that they are taking part in a research study they may well change their behaviour, even if only in a small way, and as a result the project creates change in the environment being studied.

When you read a research report it is normally quite easy to decide if the project used experimental or naturalistic methodologies. But you should also consider the extent to which an experimental study managed to control all the variables affecting it, or how much change a naturalistic project created within the environment it was studying. We will consider these research problems in more detail in Chapter 5.

## METHOD

### Quantitative or qualitative?

Most researchers seem comfortable with the idea that there are two types of research method, with the use of both types in a single study sometimes being seen as a third type, the 'mixed methods' approach. I don't view mixed methods as a separate type of research method and won't be considering it as such. To my mind, the term 'mixed methods' suggests that quantitative and qualitative methods are combined together in a way that creates a completely new approach to collecting or analysing data, when in fact what happens in practice is simply that qualitative and quantitative methods are used in the same study but remain separate. The use of both methods in a single study is a sensible approach to take, but they are not really mixed.

The difference between the two types of research method is, at one level, simple and straightforward.

- A quantitative method collects data that can be expressed as numbers and analysed using statistical tests.
- A qualitative method collects and analyses non-numerical data. It does so through the 'systematic collection, organisation, and interpretation of textual material derived from talk or observation' (Malterud, 2001, p.483).

The situation is complicated by the fact that the quantitative and qualitative methods can both be subdivided into a whole range of methods. Neale *et al* (2005, p.1585) suggest that 'qualitative' is an 'umbrella term' covering a variety of methods and the same thing can also be said of 'quantitative'. So under each umbrella we can find more-specialist methods such as surveys, interviews and others.

The umbrella covers three areas of method in particular, each of which has a variety of different ways of approaching it (remember Brechin and Sidell's identification of 15 different methods, which we noted earlier in this chapter?). These three areas are:

1   recruitment and selection;
2   data collection;
3   data analysis.

We will return to each one in later chapters.

## 'Mixed' is not the same as 'equal'

You might think that a 'mixed methods' approach to research would give equal importance to qualitative and quantitative methods, seeing each set of methods as the same in terms of their **reliability** or value to the research process. But you will only rarely find a research report in which quantitative and qualitative methods are used equally. 'Mixed methods' does not mean '50% quantitative and 50% qualitative'.

### KEY CASE 1

A well-designed research project will use the most appropriate mix of quantitative and qualitative methods, and the most appropriate mix is rarely, if ever, 50:50. An open perspective means that the researchers will consider all the different methods at their disposal and choose the best combination for dealing with their research question, but those researchers who are convinced that one specific method is the best will be less likely to be flexible. These examples show both perspectives:

* *Example 1* If I want to know the mean, or average, height of 18-year-old health and social care students in Manchester I can't think of any qualitative methods that would be of use to me. So the best mix for my needs will be 100:0 – a completely quantitative study.
* *Example 2* If I am going to study what these 18-year-old students think or feel about being the height they are, then I will probably interview them, or ask them to keep diaries, or both, then transcribe their responses and use qualitative methods to analyse them. In that case the mix will be 0:100 – a completely qualitative study.

In my first example, I think this is a perfectly acceptable approach. I am interested in the mean height of a group of people. I don't want to know what individuals think about being average, or below average, or above average height. I have no interest in their experiences of being 160 cm tall, or 185 cm tall. I just want to calculate mean height. I have considered all possible methods available to me, and decided that quantitative methods will do the job. I've taken an open perspective. But will these results be of any practical use to a health or social care practitioner?

In the second example I don't think I can produce a good-quality study, one that would be of practical use to health and social care professionals or lecturers or researchers, by using only qualitative methods. In this case, I think I was too focused on qualitative methods and was blind to the possibilities of combining methods.

My results might be more useful if I link students' subjective data, about their thoughts and feelings, with objective numerical data about their heights and weights. Do very tall females feel differently than very tall males about their height? Do these students feel more comfortable about their height if they have a normal Body Mass Index? Do short physiotherapy students feel differently about their height than do short social work students?

## TOOLS

Research tools can be thought of as the basic pieces of equipment needed to undertake a research project. Research tools can be very simple: a pad of paper and a pen are all that is needed to create a research diary, a coin may be the only tool used to allocate subjects to **intervention groups** or **control groups** in a clinical trial. Tools can also be extremely complex. The Statistical Package for the Social Sciences (SPSS) or N-Vivo are examples of software packages that can perform extremely sophisticated analysis methods.

The key to the selection of a research tool is straightforward: a tool should be used because it helps to make the process *easier*. The simplest tool that enables the job to be done is generally the best tool for the job. If my research analysis involves the use of basic mathematical techniques such as the calculation of percentages or means then a relatively simple software package such as Microsoft Excel will do the job. In fact, a basic calculator might be all I need. On the other hand, if I want to calculate statistics such as **odds ratios** or **correlations** then I will need to use a more complex package such as SPSS. Similarly, if I am using **thematic analysis** to investigate the results of five brief interviews it might be more efficient to do so using paper and pen than to spend time entering the data into a software package for analysis.

Figure 1 shows you my classification in a diagrammatic form.

## Key Question 2: What would your choices be?

If you were designing research studies to investigate the following issues, what choices of methodology, methods and tools might you make?

- Studying how effective a new surgical procedure is at curing shoulder injuries.
- Deciding which of two new social work practices with young single parents is the more cost-effective.
- Finding out what the population of a market town think about a new day centre for people with learning disabilities.

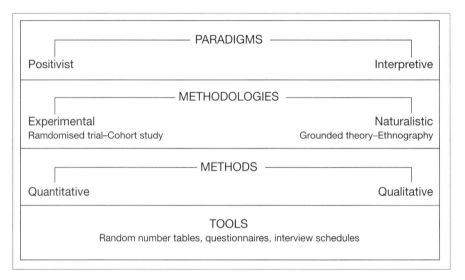

**Figure 1** Levels of choice

## THE RESEARCH HIERARCHIES

We have discussed the importance of using the most appropriate methods for an individual study and I have hopefully shown that this can be done. But you will find, as you read textbooks and research reports, that there is still a great deal of debate in health and social care research about the 'best' methods to choose. One of the most interesting parts of this debate is the idea of a research hierarchy.

A research hierarchy is a league table of research methodologies. A hierarchy proposes that certain research methodologies produce better-quality evidence than others: in other words, that the evidence they produce is more reliable than the evidence produced using methodologies from further down the list.

Research hierarchies come in two basic types, which I will call 'positivist' and 'combined'. The positivist hierarchy is a league table of research methods that are most closely associated with the positivist paradigm and the experimental methodologies. There are many versions of the positivist hierarchy but they are all essentially in agreement. Figure 2 is my version of this hierarchy. You might also want to consider other versions.

Systematic review
Randomised controlled trials
Quasi-experimental studies
Non-systematic literature reviews
Expert opinion

**Figure 2** A positivist research hierarchy

If you support this league-table approach, as many researchers do, then it provides you with clear direction in choosing a research methodology. Your first choice would be the **systematic review**. If this is not possible, because there is insufficient existing evidence, or because this evidence is of poor quality, then the next choice would be a **randomised controlled trial**. If the subject could not be studied using this method then the researcher would move on to the next level down, and so on.

Researchers who favour naturalistic methodologies do not normally view them in this hierarchical way, preferring instead to choose methods according to the research question or aim. In fact, I have not found one example of a naturalistic research hierarchy. You can think of naturalistic methodologies as appearing along a horizontal continuum, rather than a vertical hierarchy (see Figure 3).

Grounded theory – Phenomenology – Ethnography – Action research – Survey

**Figure 3** An integrative research continuum

The second type of research hierarchy, the combined hierarchy, puts experimental and naturalistic methodologies into a single league table. This causes even more concern among interpretive researchers, because most published combined hierarchies put all naturalistic methodologies below the experimental ones: they see naturalistic methodologies as 'second division'. This is a perspective that is guaranteed to cause controversy among naturalistic researchers, even though it usually creates agreement among experimental researchers.

## EXTERNAL INFLUENCES

Decisions about the design of a research project cannot be taken in isolation: they are affected by influences that are independent of a researcher's own ideas, beliefs and preferences. These influences can be so strong that they exert the most powerful effect on the design.

### Social and professional pressures

Health and social care are always in the news and are routinely seen as major political issues by politicians, professionals and the general public. However, the specific topics of concern vary with time. At the time of writing this chapter the leading health and social care topics in the UK press include obesity, hospital-acquired infections, the provision of social care in the home and the rehabilitation of offenders. If these topics continue to dominate the news it is quite likely that we will see an upsurge in research projects about them.

Social and professional pressures will have a major role in creating this upsurge. These topics are seen as critical health and social care problems and the public and politicians look to researchers for solutions. The subjects become 'high profile'. Government bodies, professional organisations and voluntary groups view them as a priority. This in turn leads researchers to focus on the subjects, in part because they, too, want solutions but also because high-profile research topics are more likely to attract funding and successful high-profile projects are likely to benefit the reputations and promotion prospects of the researchers.

### Funding bodies

Organisations that fund health and social care research will seldom, if ever, be interested in funding projects irrespective of their subjects or their research methods. If a research team hopes to attract funding, especially large grants, they are likely to be influenced in their choice of research aim and project design by the likelihood of obtaining funding. Funding organisations might set conditions on many aspects of research design, including the choice of methodology, the types of subjects or participants to be recruited, the presentation of findings and the way in which the research findings can be made public.

The amount of funding obtained will also impact on study design. If no money can be found then designs will be severely limited or, in the worst case, projects may have to be abandoned. We will discuss funding in more detail in Chapter 4.

## Research projects as a requirement for a qualification

As we have already seen, much health and social care research is under-taken in order to gain a qualification. The criteria applied to these research projects are some of the most restrictive of all. Word limits will be imposed on the final dissertation or thesis: typically around 10,000 words for a first degree (BA/BSc) to around 90,000 to 100,000 words for a PhD thesis. This has direct implications for the size of the research study. In addition, first-degree and masters projects might be restricted in terms of the type of research that can be undertaken. These criteria put clear boundaries around what is possible, but this can be helpful as it removes the need for the student personally to set these limits.

## MAKING THE FINAL CHOICE

Decisions at each of these levels are made by every researcher or research team. Some decisions might be quick and simple, others may be long and complicated. Occasionally the decisions are made by someone else: for example, an organisation may pay for a project but insist that it be carried out in a particular way. What is important for researchers and users of research to realise is that in health and social care these decisions always have alternatives. Whatever decisions are taken in the creation of a research project, at one or more levels an alternative could have been chosen.

Unless a researcher has unlimited time, money and resources the final choice of research design is going to be a compromise between what the researcher would ideally like to do and what is achievable. A high propor-tion of health and social care research is small-scale, often severely time-limited and carried out without financial support. As a result, the researcher has to accept major constraints on the design. Even large-scale, well-funded and well-resourced projects have some limitations. As a potential user of research findings you need to be aware of this and to take these limitations into account when judging the quality of a piece of research. I will discuss this further in Chapter 7. In Chapter 4 we will con-sider the issues of research costs and research ethics.

KEY LEARNING POINTS

- The design of a research project results from a series of decisions.
- The researcher's beliefs about knowledge and understanding (the paradigm) lead to decisions about the best ways of designing research studies (the methodology), which lead to decisions about the best ways of collecting and analysing data (the method), which lead to decisions about the tools that are needed.
- Research hierarchies can be positivist or combined. The positivist hierarchies are widely supported and used. The combined hierarchies are more contentious and often opposed, particularly by qualitative researchers.
- Research design is also affected by external factors, such as the amount of money available to the research team, or the time available. These limitations affect the extent to which the researcher's ideal design can be put into practice.

## FURTHER READING

Grbich, C (2007) *Qualitative data analysis. An introduction*. London: Sage

Holliday, A (2007) *Doing and writing qualitative research* (2nd edn). London: Sage

Malterud, K (2001) 'Qualitative research: standards, challenges, and guidelines'. *The Lancet*, 358: 483–8

Medical Research Council (2005) *Good research practice. MRC ethics series*. London: MRC

In addition, try to read research papers from a variety of different journals and on a variety of different health and social care subjects. The more papers you read the easier it will become to appraise and review them.

# Chapter 4

# Can It Be Done? Funding and Ethics

This chapter discusses the following topics.

- Who funds research?

- How much does research cost?

- How is research funding allocated?

- What ethical issues are important?

- Gaining ethical approval for research.

## INTRODUCTION

In Chapter 3, I discussed the internal factors that result in the development of a research project. Towards the end of the chapter I also discussed the idea that most projects are constrained by limits on resources. In this chapter I want to expand this discussion with regard to two major issues in health and social care research. These issues are research funding and research ethics. Every health and social care research project is affected by these two factors.

Research costs money. I'm sure that you are aware of this, but you are probably less aware of exactly how much money. In this chapter I will discuss the costs of research, who pays for it and how money is allocated. You may not feel that knowing about research funding will be of much help to you in judging the usefulness of research findings, but I disagree. Knowing the cost of research and the way in which funding is allocated helps you to understand why some research methods are less expensive than others, why so many health and social care research projects are small-scale and even why some subjects seem over-researched while others seem under-researched.

Health and social care research must be of good quality to be useful to practitioners. But it is also the case that this research must be ethical. The rights and wrongs of research using animals or human embryos are regularly debated in the media, but most ethical issues in health and social care are on a much smaller scale, although they are no less important. Potential issues are wide-ranging, covering factors such as risk, consent and benefit. No research project involving human subjects or participants should take place unless it has been assessed and found to be ethically satisfactory. In the UK and other countries this usually involves submitting the research proposal to an ethics committee for its approval. Later in this chapter I will discuss ethical issues and the ethics approval process.

## WHO FUNDS RESEARCH?

Large projects are impossible to undertake without dedicated funding. Health and social care research is paid for by four main funding sources. These are:

- European or national government (including the European Community and government departments such as the Department of Health);
- local or national government-funded organisations (in particular the NHS, local councils and the Research Councils);
- voluntary or charitable organisations (such as the Rowntree Foundation and the Wellcome Trust);
- commercial companies.

The proportion of funds provided by each of these sources varies from country to country and from subject to subject, but each one makes substantial contributions to health and social care research. Of course, in the case of central government and government-funded organisations, the money comes from the taxpayer and in the case of commercial companies it comes from the profits generated by sales, so it is true to say that research is actually funded by you and me.

## Allocating research funds

Researchers gain funding in three main ways:

1 the researcher develops an idea, writes a proposal and then submits it to an appropriate funding organisation;
2 a funding organisation decides to commission research on a specific topic or theme and advertises for researchers to submit applications;
3 researchers are approached specifically by a funding organisation and asked to undertake a project. This is an unusual way to gain funds, usually open only to researchers with strong international reputations.

Most researchers will try to gain funding through the first or second of these methods. Health and social care research is extremely competitive however, and most funding organisations receive more applications than they can fund. In 2005–2006, for example, the Economic and Social Research Council (ESRC) received 1001 applications for research grants and funded 272, a funding rate of 27%.

## Prestige and funding

You might think that money is money and so the source of research funds is irrelevant. But funding, like many other issues in health and social care research, is more complicated than that. Some sources of research funds are considered to be more prestigious than others, while some researchers view certain sources of funds with concern.

### Key Question 1

If you were looking for a large amount of money to fund a project would you have concerns about taking money from certain sources? If so, what might your concerns be?

In the UK, for example, the Research Councils are viewed as particularly prestigious sources of funds, especially by university-based researchers. By contrast, many researchers are reluctant to apply for funding from commercial organisations such as pharmaceutical companies, medical equipment manufacturers or cigarette makers. These researchers are concerned about the conditions that such funders might place on the use of findings or about the ways in which the companies make their profits, or are worried that research funded in this way will be seen as **biased** or lacking independence. This mistrust of some sources of research funds can be extreme. Research sponsorship by tobacco manufacturers is a good example, with many researchers possibly holding the same opinion as Chapman and Shatenstein (2001, p.1) that: 'The tobacco industry … has hung about university research funding corridors like a wheel of ripe cheese in a sun-baked phone booth …'.

### Key Question 2

Can you think of any possible sources of bias in the funding of these projects?

- A study of the effects of smoking, paid for by a multi-national tobacco company.
- A small study of the quality of care in a residential home, paid for by the company that owns the home.
- A study of stress in health workers, paid for by a leading health service trade union.

# HOW MUCH DOES RESEARCH COST?

In 2004 the gross expenditure on research and development in the UK was £21 billion (National Statistics, 2006). It is difficult to tell what proportion of this spending was on health and social care research, but the figure is probably well over 10%. We can get some idea of the money spent on health and social care research from the following examples. The Department of Health's budget for research in 2006–2007 was £753 million (Department of Health, 2007). The Medical Research Council's expenditure in 2005–2006 was £510 million, spread across 851 research grants (MRC, 2006).

If we think of a specific research project then the cost could be anything from a few hundred pounds to a few million. But research is never 'free'. You might often read reports that state that the research was unfunded, but that does not mean that it cost nothing. All research projects have a cost.

## The cost of a research project

### Key Question 3

How much do you think it would cost to run each of the following types of project?

- A large **randomised controlled trial** of a new drug.
- A survey of 1000 social workers using a postal questionnaire.
- An interview-based study of ten midwives from across the UK.
- A **systematic review** of research into the admission of patients to hospital.

Here are some recent research projects and their costs:

- 'Refugees and the law: An ethnography of the British asylum system' – awarded £483,001 in July 2006 by the ESRC;
- 'Vocal and non-vocal communication in autism' – awarded £151,000 by the MRC;
- 'Carers - Measuring outcomes for carers for people with mental health problems' – awarded £74,053 by the NHS Service Delivery and Organisation Programme (NHS SDO);
- 'Educating nurses to meet the emotional and psychological needs of hospitalised children' – awarded £1500 by the Wellcome Foundation.

As you can see, costs vary considerably from project to project. The costs vary for many reasons, including the type and length of the study, the number of subjects or participants and the complexity of the data collection and analysis methods. When researchers are developing projects they need to be able to calculate accurately the costs before being awarded the funds to carry the project out. These costs are divided across different aspects of the project, four of which I will now discuss.

## Staff costs

In health and social care research this is one of the largest areas of expenditure. A medium- or large-scale research project will probably employ one or more junior researchers to undertake the bulk of the work. The senior researcher in charge of the project, often referred to as the Principal Investigator, is unlikely to work on it full time, but will allocate one or two days a week to its management. There is likely to be administrative support from another member of staff, whose time must also be paid for. As well as the salaries of staff a research grant will also need to pay the 'on-costs' relating to employer's tax, National Insurance and pension contributions.

## Equipment and related costs

Funders of health and social care research rarely pay for standard equipment such as telephones or desktop computers. If a project needs specialist pieces of equipment, such as specific computer software or audio or video recorders, then these costs might be included in the grant. Related costs such as paper, envelopes or postage will also need to be included.

## Travel

Some projects can involve large amounts of national or international travel and the costs of mileage, rail tickets or flights and accommodation can add up to thousands of pounds. Researchers might also plan to present their work at conferences and the cost of conference fees and accommodation can also be substantial.

## Payments to subjects or participants

In some areas of research it's usual to pay participants or subjects. In Phase 1 clinical trials, when new drugs are tested on healthy volunteers in projects that may require the subjects to commit a period of weeks exclusively to the study, the payments may be hundreds or thousands of pounds. In the health and social care research projects that we are concerned about in this book, this level of payment is not reached. In fact, health and social care researchers in the UK do not usually offer payments to participants at all. Expenses are routinely reimbursed, while a small amount of money might also be given when the research involves some effort on the part of the participants, for example in varying their eating habits or in completing a diary over a period of time. Payments in excess of these small sums are discouraged.

## 'Unfunded' research

The proportion of health and social care research projects that receive no outside funding, often somewhat incorrectly referred to as 'unfunded' projects, is high (Lindsay *et al*, 2001). As a result, the true cost of research is hidden. Research projects do not always gain funds from outside sources, but they always have a cost.

What types of research are done without external funding? Small-scale studies, carried out in a practitioner's own workplace or undertaken as part of a course, are commonly undertaken without external funding and can be very successful. Research studies for undergraduate courses, masters degrees and even PhDs are often undertaken without external funding. So, too, are many **pilot studies** in preparation for full-scale projects, as well as many literature reviews and exploratory studies. Talk to students or practitioners who are undertaking research on this basis and they will routinely say things such as 'I'm doing it on my days off, so it doesn't cost anything' or 'I'm using the PC at work and the department secretary prints out the questionnaires and posts them so I don't need funding'. But the work still needs funding from somewhere.

As an example, let's take the second quote and assume that this researcher is using a questionnaire to gather data for a small project, using equipment and staff at work to help with the study. If we assume that the questionnaire took a few hours to design, during work time and on work equipment, the hidden costs begin to emerge:

- the researcher's 'design time' during working hours;
- the researcher's time outside working hours – this also has a value, even if it isn't easily calculated in monetary terms;
- costs of the PC – electricity, wear and tear;
- the secretary's wages for 'printing and posting' time;
- costs of printing – paper, laser cartridge;
- costs of postage (stamps, envelopes).

The 'free' and 'unfunded' research project hides its costs within the general departmental budget. The individual project may not be expensive – the example above might cost a few hundred pounds – but if four or five small projects are carried out by every directorate or team every year the total cost to an NHS Trust or a Social Services Department can be substantial.

Research costs money. Even small-scale projects have a financial cost and eventually this cost must be met, whether it's by researchers giving their own time to a project or by means of a large grant from a government department or a commercial company. If no-one is willing to meet the costs of a study then it doesn't get done. If a research project is carried out then this is because someone has, at some stage, made the decision that the project is worth doing. But this is not the only decision that has to be made in order for a project to begin. There should also be a decision about the ethical nature of the project.

## ETHICAL ISSUES IN HEALTH AND SOCIAL CARE RESEARCH

In health and social care all research projects must be ethical. In other words, they must conform to acceptable standards of practice and conduct (National Health and Medical Research Council of Australia, 1999). Some projects, for example systematic reviews using data gathered from publicly-available documents, have few if any ethical concerns. Most projects in health and social care are less straightforward and require formal ethical approval. Researchers must always consider ethical issues when planning projects and no project should go ahead unless ethical approval has been gained.

## WHAT ARE THE ETHICAL ISSUES?

- When is research acceptable and when is it not?
- Whose well-being should take priority: a research subject's or that of the population as a whole?
- Is it okay to lie to a research subject, to recruit people against their will, to carry out experiments that carry a high risk of death or injury?
- Is it acceptable to use clients' or patients' records for research without gaining their permission?
- Are ethical issues the same across all health and social care research, all countries and all cultures, all social groups?

All of the above questions are ethical questions. They are questions about the 'rights' and 'wrongs' of research design and research practice. The list is not intended to be exhaustive and I do not intend to answer all those questions in this book. Indeed, as you will see, many questions about research ethics are still being debated: we haven't yet decided exactly what is 'right' or 'wrong' in health and social care research. It is important for you to ask these questions as a potential user of research findings, as a potential participant or subject in a research study and also as a potential researcher yourself.

### When did people start worrying about ethics in research?

The Second World War is viewed by writers such as Benatar (2004) as the event which stimulated concern about the ethics of research. Experiments carried out on human beings by scientists working for the Nazi government created revulsion when they were brought to light and in 1947 the Nuremberg Code was formulated (Antle and Regehr, 2003). More recently,

codes for the undertaking of health and social care research have prolifer-
ated. The Declaration of Helsinki (World Medical Association, 2004)
remains one of the most influential of these. The Declaration, produced
originally in 1964 and amended on seven occasions since then, focuses on
medical research involving human subjects. A Code of Ethics for social
work and social care research has also been developed (Butler, 2002).

Concerns about research ethics and attempts to develop ethical codes and
frameworks for research practice in health and social care have certainly
expanded in the last few decades, but this does not mean that researchers
were not concerned about ethics before the Second World War. Rather,
research ethics were less of a priority and what was considered to be ethically acceptable was in many respects different from today.

Ethical questions are often complex and presented in ways that can make
them difficult, if not impossible, to understand. Solomon Benatar (2004)
suggests that the debate regarding research ethics occurs on two levels: the
practical and the theoretical. At the practical level the controversy is about
'… the competing concerns of those predominantly interested in doing
research to advance knowledge and those who, while supporting the need
for research, are more acutely aware of the potential to exploit vulnerable
participants …' (p.574). At the theoretical level the debate 'pits ethical
universalism against moral relativism' (p.574): in other words, a belief in a
set of principles that apply everywhere and in all circumstances versus a
belief that ideas of right and wrong can change according to circumstances. So how might these practical and theoretical issues affect health
and social care research and its impact on practice?

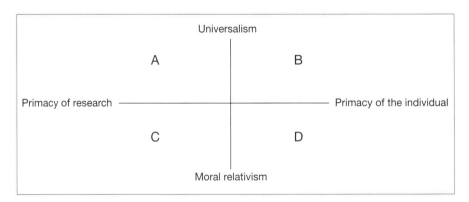

**Figure 1**

Figure 1 is my interpretation of Benatar's argument. In Figure 1 the letters
A, B, C and D represent different perspectives on Benatar's ethical ten-
sions. Each one has the potential to create a very different ethical climate
within which research might take place.

**A:** *A belief in the primacy of research and in the universality of ethics* This combination of beliefs, putting the search for evidence above the rights of individuals, could lead to a society that sees as acceptable the compulsory participation of individuals in research studies without their consent and without concern for the risk they are exposed to.

**B:** *A belief in the primacy of the individual and in the universality of ethics* This combination again sees ethics as constant, but puts people first. This could create an approach to research where the individual always has the right to refuse to take part in research, even where such research would be of benefit to the human race as a whole and would not put that individual at risk.

**C:** *A belief in the primacy of research and in moral relativism* With this combination a society could view the compulsory participation of individuals without their consent as acceptable in certain circumstances: when the individual is a criminal, perhaps, or when the predicted contribution to knowledge is seen as great enough to take precedence over individual rights.

**D:** *A belief in moral relativism and in the primacy of the individual* This mix of beliefs could view the individual's right to refuse to participate in research as a key right, unless circumstances were such that this refusal could be damaging to the well-being of society as a whole.

## Key Question 4

Where would you put yourself in Figure 1? How might your ethical beliefs affect your approach to carrying out research, taking part in a project or using research findings?

[I think I'm probably a 'D', while current thinking in health and social care probably favours B.]

## An ethical code for both health and social care?

In England the Department of Health published its *Research Governance Framework for Health and Social Care* in 2005. In this document the government made it clear that it supported the idea of a single set of guiding principles for both fields of research. The document describes **research governance** as a system which:

- sets out principles, requirements and standards for research;
- defines mechanisms to deliver these principles, requirements and standards;
- improves research and safeguards the public.

The same principles of governance apply across health and social care, according to the document, but the achievement of these standards will vary according to the exact nature of the research design. The application of research ethics is part of this over-arching research governance framework.

Current debate in the academic press suggests that health and social care researchers favour a relativist approach to research ethics. The writers, especially those from social care, support the idea that many of the ethical issues in health research differ from those in social care research and that research ethics should therefore be treated differently across the disciplines.

Butler (2002) sums up this professional relativism when justifying the need for a code of practice specific to social work and social care research. Codes of ethics, according to Butler (p.240), 'are not for always and for everywhere … they inevitably articulate the occupational/professional, ideological and moral aspirations of their creators.' Miller (2004), in his discussion of medicine, proposes that research and care are significantly ethically different and so we should not judge the conduct of research according to the same standards we would use to judge care.

Other writers suggest that research ethics differ according to the chosen research paradigm, or the preferred methodology, or the cultural context in which research occurs. Sanders (2003, p.113) proposes that the ethical approval process developed for medical research is 'often wholly inappropriate' for social work researchers because medical research focuses heavily on **randomised controlled trials** while social care research uses **ethnographic** approaches. By contrast, Antle and Regehr (2003) contrast health care and social care research ethics but argue in favour of both disciplines adopting the same basic approach to ethical codes and procedures, adapting this approach to meet the specific needs of each body of researchers.

Shaw (2003) argues in favour of developing ethical codes and approval processes based on the different ethical issues raised by different research paradigms or methodologies. Both Shaw and Sanders appear to lack a clear understanding of medical/health care research and also to have a rather compartmentalised view of research design. Shaw, for example, seems not to understand that randomised controlled trials can include qualitative methods of data collection and analysis. Such a lack of understanding weakens both their arguments and in turn weakens their support of separate ethical approaches. The MRC (2005), in contrast, has developed its *Good Research Practice* guidance with a clear emphasis on positivist, quantitative, research. This lack of recognition of interpretative, qualitative, research is guaranteed to antagonise and upset those researchers working with these approaches.

You also need to be aware that while a recognition of the need for ethical research appears to be almost universal this is not the same as saying that research ethics are universal. Different countries can have different ideas about the major ethical issues in research, or about how ethical approval is given and on what grounds. Even focusing just on Europe we can easily find examples of differences in research ethics. In France, less emphasis is placed on individual consent by research participants than in the UK or Germany, but therapeutic benefit is considered to be a more important issue (Maio, 2002). The emphasis on formal ethical approval also varies. Hearnshaw (2004) investigated the need for ethical approval for a study of information leaflets to help older people improve their interactions with their doctors. She compared the process in eleven European countries and found that eight countries did not require formal approval by an ethics committee, because the study was considered non-invasive. Three countries did require formal approval: Belgium, Slovenia and the UK. In Slovenia approval took two days to be granted, in the UK it took ten weeks.

Another concern voiced by many naturalistic researchers relates to what Haggerty (2004) calls ethics creep. This refers to the expansion of the need for formal ethical approval into more and more areas of study. Early ethical approval processes were designed to protect subjects from risk during invasive projects. Current Central Office of Research Ethics Committees (COREC) guidelines state that approval is needed from NHS ethics committees if research involves staff or patients even where the research is non-invasive, while university ethics committees are being expanded to deal with an ever-increasing range of research projects which only a few years ago would not have needed to gain ethical approval.

## KEY CASE 1

This expansion of the scope and power of ethics approval processes reflects society's own move from an assumption that researchers are competent and responsible to an assumption that they lack the ability to control their own activities (Haggerty, 2004). In contrast, journalists undertake research on a daily basis without the need to subject their planned activities to formal ethical scrutiny. If you think of naturalistic research methodologies, using observation and interview to collect data and **thematic analysis** to make sense of it, you can see how closely they resemble the journalist's processes for collecting information and producing a report. So why does the 'researcher' have to go through a rigorous approval process when a journalist does not?

## GAINING ETHICAL APPROVAL

While there is still a great deal of debate about research ethics in health and social care, in recent years broad agreement has been reached about one thing: health and social care research projects should gain ethical approval before they begin. This agreement about the need for ethical approval leads to another unusual and somewhat puzzling practical issue. Health and social care researchers need to gain ethical approval, but the process by which such approval is gained, the organisations and individuals granting the approval, the ethical issues under consideration and the complexities of the process vary across disciplines, countries and institutions.

Any research paper published in the last few years should, as a matter of good practice, state that ethical approval for the project was gained (or should make it clear why such approval was not necessary). You can then, as a reader and a potential user of the findings, be confident that the research design met the required ethical standards. What is harder to establish, however, is exactly what those standards were. This is particularly the case if the study was designed and undertaken in another country, or in a discipline with which you are unfamiliar.

## READING RESEARCH – IDENTIFYING ETHICAL ISSUES

When you are reading a research report, try to identify the ethical issues for the project yourself. Many ethical issues are also practical issues. Other ethical issues are more abstract or theoretical, but just as important. Remember also that while ethical approval supports the relevance and validity of the research it is not an absolute guarantee of the quality of the research.

Specific ethical issues vary from project to project, but you will find that the following apply to most research.

- *Appropriateness* – should this project take place? Is it necessary?
- *Consent* – will all participants or subjects be able to give **informed consent**? If not, should they be recruited? If they should be, who can give permission for their participation?
- *Participant/subject safety* – is there a risk to the well-being of the people taking part? How big is the risk? Is risk outweighed by potential benefits?
- *Researcher safety* – is there a risk to the members of the research team? How can it be minimised?
- *Bias* – this exists in every research project, but is it an unethical bias?

When you read a research report you might well find that you have concerns about the ethics of the study. Identify your concerns clearly, then try to think about why these issues might not have been seen as problematic by the researchers or by the ethics committee that gave approval, assuming such approval was given. As we have noted, research ethics is not an exact science and there is no simple list of ethical 'rights' and 'wrongs' that can be universally applied.

---

### KEY LEARNING POINTS

- Research costs money: even so-called 'unfunded research'.
- The amount of money available to an individual research project greatly impacts on its potential design, size and scope.
- The source of research funds can be of ethical concern.
- Ethical approval, or clear proof that approval is unnecessary, is needed for any research projects that involve human subjects, especially if they are vulnerable or the project carries actual or potential risk.

---

## FURTHER READING

Benatar, SR (2004) 'Towards progress in resolving dilemmas in international research ethics'. *Journal of Law, Medicine and Ethics*, 32: 574–82

Butler, I (2002) 'A code of ethics for social work and social care research'. *British Journal of Social Work*, 32: 239–48

Department of Health (2005) *Research governance framework for health and social care*. London: Department of Health. This is a key policy document that has helped to shape research practice in health and social care.

Department of Health (2007) *Research funding and priorities*. **www.dh.gov.uk/en/Policyandguidance/Researchanddevelopment/A-Z/DH_4069152** (20 June 2007)

Medical Research Council (2005) *Good research practice. MRC ethics series*. London: MRC

Shaw, IF (2003) 'Ethics in qualitative research and evaluation'. *Journal of Social Work*, 3: 9–29

World Medical Association (2004) *Declaration of Helsinki. World Medical Association*. **www.wma.net/e/policy/pdf/17c.pdf** (February 2007). This is one of the most influential documents in health care research and a good example of how a policy document can still be relevant nearly 50 years after it was originally written.

**Chapter 5**

# Recruitment and Data Collection

This chapter discusses how to recruit to a study and gather data.

- Developing inclusion and exclusion criteria.

- Selection and sampling issues.

- Randomisation and allocation.

- Obtaining consent.

- The impact of rewards.

- Major data collection issues – blinding, Hawthorne Effect, honesty.

- Data storage – confidentiality and anonymity.

## INTRODUCTION

The study has been designed, enough money has been found to pay for it and ethical approval has been given. A detailed literature review has been carried out. So far, so good. The next step is to recruit enough participants or subjects for the study: a process that can run smoothly and lead to a meaningful and useful project or a process that can be so problematic that it can lead to the collapse of the entire study.

Once recruitment has been carried out data collection can begin. This, too, is a process that appears straightforward but can become a lengthy and frustrating activity which fails to meet the study's needs. Both recruitment and data collection are often overlooked by students when they attempt to critique or assess research papers because they are seen as less important and less complex than data analysis. But effective analysis demands effective data and this is not obtained unless the process of gathering data is sound. This process begins with the identification of the data sources: in health and social care research, the subjects or participants. It goes on to encompass the design of data collection tools and activities, which is crucial to the quality of data for analysis.

## RECRUITMENT ISSUES

Health and social care research studies people, but very little health and social care research is interested in 'people in general'. Instead, we are interested in studying defined groups of individuals who share some characteristics but not others. We may be interested in men but not women, children but not adults, people who have diabetes but not asthma, or people with asthma but not diabetes. The recruitment of the 'right' group of people is crucial for the success of a research project. Unfortunately for the researcher and for the potential user of findings there is no single way of recruiting to a study and no single definition of the 'right' set of subjects or participants. Experimental and naturalistic methodologies each have their own broad sets of guidelines or expectations for recruitment and data collection, which are refined further in individual project designs. We will now discuss some of the major issues in the recruitment process.

## PARTICIPANTS OR SUBJECTS?

In health and social care research we can study cells, or organs, or animals. But most of the health and social care research of direct relevance to practice studies people and refers to those people as subjects or participants. Sometimes researchers use these words interchangeably, but it is more useful to see them as having slightly different meanings.

As a very general rule positivist researchers refer to subjects and interpretative researchers talk about participants. 'Subject' suggests a passive role in research, where the individual has something done to them and has little if any influence on how the research progresses. In a typical **randomised controlled trial**, for example, a drug or a control substance is given to each subject and 'objective' outcome measures such as biochemical or physiological changes are recorded.

'Participant' suggests a more active role for the people in the study. Participation involves more than just allowing something to happen to you. Being a participant involves making choices about your responses in an interview, or how you behave when you are being observed. **Participant corroboration** or **member checking**, where interview transcripts are shown to interviewees for comment or clarification, gives these interviewees some control over the data to be analysed.

## Key Question 1

In the following research studies, would you describe the people taking part as participants or subjects?

- A trial of a new surgical procedure, using data on wound infection rates, pre-scribed analgesic medication and lengths of hospital admissions.
- An interview-based study of clients' experiences of a day centre.
- An observational study of a child protection team: the researcher is a member of the team.
- A multi-centre study of the use of cognitive behavioural therapy, using data gathered from therapists completing structured online forms.

## DEVELOPING INCLUSION AND EXCLUSION CRITERIA

We have already discussed inclusion and exclusion criteria in relation to reviewing the literature. When developing these criteria for the recruitment of participants or subjects the same basic aim applies: to ensure that we collect data from appropriate sources and do not inadvertently gather data from inappropriate sources.

To develop effective inclusion and exclusion criteria the researcher needs to have a clear understanding of the population of interest. This should have been gained at the stage of defining the research aim and should give a clear set of characteristics that define this population. This does not mean that we need to consider every characteristic that a population might have, only those of importance to the study we wish to carry out. Key Case 1 gives some examples of criteria from the literature. As you will see, not every study makes its inclusion and exclusion criteria explicit in a formal way such as through the use of a table or bullet points, but they can be identified or at least inferred by the reader.

## KEY CASE 1 – Criteria from real studies

- Stewart *et al* (2005) used two basic criteria: any person over 65 years old referred to Cambridgeshire Social Services was considered for inclusion. Individuals were excluded from the study only if they required an urgent response from the Social Services team.
- Coren *et al* (2003) used a single inclusion criterion in their **systematic review** of home-based support for disadvantaged mothers: studies were suitable for inclusion if they assigned study participants to groups using random or quasi-random methods.

- Caplin *et al* (2006) used a Delphi Study design to identify performance indicators for managing paediatric epilepsy. They used inclusion criteria that focused on participants' expertise in epilepsy care. In addition they decided that the majority of participants needed to have current clinical responsibility.
- Paterson *et al* (2005) investigated massage for people with Parkinson's disease. Members of a branch of the Parkinson's Disease Society were selected by the branch on the basis of two inclusion criteria: their willingness to take part and their representation of a wide range of illness severity.

## SELECTION AND SAMPLING

Once the inclusion and exclusion criteria have been developed the researcher can use them in the recruitment of participants or subjects. The key question at this point is probably: 'How big is the population?'

If your research aim is to study a very specific population, located within a small geographical area for instance, then it may be possible to recruit the entire population. The aim might be to analyse the impact of a new practice on the work of probation officers in a single Scottish county, or to analyse the working patterns of staff in a new health centre in a Welsh market town. Both of these studies have well-defined populations which are easily identifiable and easily contactable. A 100% sample is theoretically possible, although, of course, not everyone might agree to take part. But what if the aim is to observe the counselling services in further education colleges in the UK? Unless the study is extremely well-resourced there are likely to be too many colleges and counselling services to study every one of them. With a study of the impact of a new drug on the blood pressures of people with hypertension the problem becomes even greater. The population is a worldwide one, with millions of potential subjects. Even the best-resourced study couldn't recruit everyone, even if it wanted to. For these last two examples the only option is to sample.

## SAMPLING

There are two or three main ways of recruiting a sample from a larger population. The right way for a particular study will depend on the nature of the sample that the study needs. Does the sample need to match the characteristics of the overall population, or does it need to include participants with particular characteristics that may not be shared by the population as a whole? If the sample needs to match the overall population then it is said to be representative and your sampling method is likely to be based on probability sampling. If you want to target specific characteristics, or if you have limitations on your freedom to recruit, then you will choose a purposive method of selection.

## The representative sample

If you have a large population that you wish to study, but you can study only a small proportion of it, you need to ensure that the sample matches, or is representative of, the overall population. To recruit a representative sample, researchers usually use a process of sampling that ensures that every member of the population has an equal chance of being invited to take part in the study. This is referred to as probability sampling. If your population has been clearly defined then those members that are recruited will be 'typical' and your sample will be representative, provided that the selection has been **randomised**.

The unbiased selection of research subjects or participants is usually seen as a crucial stage in a **positivist** research project. Positivist researchers go to great lengths to ensure the unbiased nature of this process by sampling or selecting in a randomised way. True randomisation gives everyone within a population the same chance of being selected for a project and also ensures that no-one in the research team can influence this recruitment process.

In some populations a variation of randomisation may be necessary to create a representative sample. This variation involves **stratification**. In stratified random sampling the total population is subdivided into groups, or strata, according to characteristics that are seen as potentially important to the study. If the population divides neatly into groups of similar size then stratification is fairly simple. If gender is the characteristic of importance and a population consists of 50% males and 50% females then the research team can select half their sample from each group. If the groups or strata are not of equal size then the sample needs to maintain these unequal proportions. This is referred to as weighting.

## The purposive sample

Not every research project seeks a representative or random sample. Some studies will target specific individuals within a population, or will select people with particular characteristics, or will be unable to recruit a representative sample. In those cases **purposive sampling** can be used. In this form of sampling the research team deliberately select their participants because they have specific characteristics: as Green and Thorogood (2004, p.102) put it, the team are 'explicitly selecting interviewees who it is intended will generate appropriate data'.

There are at least 15 separate methods of purposive sampling in the literature. Some are more objective than others: some are deliberately intended to introduce a **bias** to the study. Others are simply ways of explaining selection processes that are primarily intended to make the researcher's life easy, or to overcome problems that obstruct the use of more reliable methods (although not every researcher believes that these approaches are actually purposive).

## Types of purposive sampling

- Snowball sampling (also known as chain sampling): the first participant in a study is asked to identify other members of the population who may be suitable for inclusion. This is useful for accessing hard-to-reach groups or groups that may be suspicious of outsiders.
- Maximum variation sampling: study participants are selected to ensure that they vary as widely as possible. This variation could be, for example, by age, length of experience, household income or any other relevant characteristic.
- Case sampling: a series of 'cases' or events are selected to be studied in depth as a way of understanding the overall situation or phenomenon. Case sampling may be of 'typical' cases which represent average or run-of-the-mill activity, 'extreme' cases which represent the most unusual events or phenomena, or 'critical' cases which are seen as the most important cases for an understanding of the phenomenon.
- Convenience sampling: participants are chosen for the convenience of the researcher. This may involve selecting participants who live within an hour's drive of the researcher's home, or selecting from patients who attend a clinic on a Thursday because this is the only day the researcher can also attend. This is generally seen as the most inefficient and unreliable method of sampling. Despite this, it is also one of the most common sampling methods in health and social care research.
- Opportunistic sampling: this takes advantage of opportunities to recruit new participants as they arise. It makes use of the flexibility of a project's design to expand the study population as the chance arises.

Definitions of purposive sampling methods are not consistent. As I noted earlier, many researchers would not class convenience or opportunistic sampling strategies as purposive, while some authors see convenience and opportunistic sampling strategies as two versions of a single approach.

## HOW BIG SHOULD THE SAMPLE BE?

Sample size is affected by research design, intended methods of data analysis, the research aim and many other factors, so there is no hard and fast answer to this question except, perhaps, 'big enough'. But this is not very helpful on its own.

Positivist studies, especially if they aim to establish a cause-and-effect relationship between variables, often apply a statistical method known as **power calculation** to assess how large the study sample needs to be. This uses information about a range of criteria to identify the minimum number of subjects or participants a study needs in order for it to produce statistically significant results. Stewart *et al* (2005), for example, used a power calculation based on the need to be able to identify clinically important differences in participant scores in the Community Dependency Index to identify the need to recruit at least 300 individuals to their study.

Within the relativist paradigm each methodology appears to have its own ideas about sample size. These ideas are based not on power calculations but on factors ranging from pragmatic criteria, such as how much data can be collected within the study's resources, to more theoretical criteria, such as **grounded theory's** concept of data saturation. This concept refers to the way in which data is collected in grounded theory studies. In most studies the research team decide in advance how large the study population will be. In grounded theory recruitment continues until no new information is being received: in other words, until the researchers are no longer identifying any new themes or concepts. At this point the data is said to be 'saturated'.

Relativism's varied approach to the question of sample size has been the focus of much criticism, especially from positivist researchers and especially of the very small numbers of participants to be found in much **phenomenological** research. But we should remember that interpretivist researchers usually seek a deep understanding of a specific situation or phenomenon and aim for thick description, while positivist researchers hope to generalise from their results. So each group samples with different aims in mind.

## KEY CASE 2 – Sampling sizes

- Wright *et al* (1998) recruited 229 children to their randomised controlled trial of community-based management of failure to thrive. This number was the result of recruiting all children diagnosed with failure to thrive within a defined geographical area and within a study period of two years.
- Caplin *et al* (2006) recruited 13 panel members (from the 16 experts who were invited to take part) in their Delphi Study on epilepsy care.
- Paterson *et al* (2005) recruited seven participants to their pilot observational study of massage for people with Parkinson 's disease.
- Stewart *et al* (2005) recruited 321 people to their randomised trial of assessments of older people. This number was based on a power calculation that identified 300 participants as the smallest number needed to give clinically significant results.

# ATTRITION

Attrition, where participants or subjects are lost to the study before they complete their intended participation, is a problem that potentially affects all health and social care research projects. Attrition rates are affected by issues such as:

- numbers of people originally recruited;
- length of the study;
- risks or benefits to the participants or subjects;
- data being collected;
- methods of data collection;
- level of subject or participant activity required.

The impact attrition can have on a study depends on the study design and on the number of participants or subjects who fail to complete their involvement. In a randomised trial an attrition rate that results in the study numbers falling below that required by the power calculation can badly affect the generalisability and **validity** of the results. In a small-scale interview-based study dropouts may have to be replaced in order to retain the overall balance of participants or, if not replaced, they may alter the balance of participants and lead to the study no longer achieving its aim. In a survey study using questionnaires attrition or non-response, as measured by the percentage of participants failing to return a completed questionnaire, may also have a strong negative impact on validity and generalisability. Gomm and Davies (2000, p.31) suggest that non-response rates above 25% in a survey 'should begin to raise suspicions about the representativeness of a sample'.

I will return to the question of dropout in Chapter 6, when we discuss data analysis.

# OBTAINING CONSENT

Before taking part in a research study individuals must give their consent in writing, by signing a consent form. This consent must be based on sufficient information about the study and about what they will be required to do: it must be **informed consent**.

There are some exceptions to this rule. In a questionnaire survey the return of the completed questionnaire is taken to be a sign of consent. Other safeguards are in place for studies involving individuals who cannot give their own consent, such as infants or unconscious patients (see, for example, Chronic Poverty Research Centre, undated). But most studies involve individuals who are able to give consent and researchers need to ensure that sufficient information is made available to individuals who are interested in participating. For projects in the UK a useful set of guidelines for information and consent forms can be found on the website of the National Research Ethics Service (NRES: **www.nres.npsa.nhs.uk**).

Not only must consent be informed, it must be freely given without the person feeling that they are being forced into taking part. In health and social care research this issue of free as well as informed consent is often a complex one and people may feel pressure to take part in a study even when no such pressure is intended.

> ## Key Question 2 – Pressure to consent?
>
> Force or coercion is not always deliberate. People can feel forced into taking part in research even when this is not the intention of the research team. How would you feel about taking part in these research projects?
>
> - **Project 1**: the Housing Association that rents you your flat sends you a questionnaire asking for your views on the quality of their service. The covering letter stresses that all responses are anonymous and your identity will not be known.
> - **Project 2**: you attend a hospital appointment with your consultant. He asks if you would like to take part in a new drug trial he is undertaking. Participation is voluntary. However he mentions, seemingly as an afterthought, that he will see only study participants in the clinic in future. All other patients will be seen by a member of the consultant's junior medical team.
> - **Project 3**: your line manager is studying for a masters qualification and needs to carry out a research project for her qualification. The project will require each participant to be interviewed three times and to spend a weekend on an 'activity break' that she refuses to describe in more detail. She asks you to take part.

## GIVING REWARDS

Another decision the researcher needs to make is whether or not to reward the participants or subjects in some way. Most research projects in the UK do not offer any incentives but some do, particularly if the participants or subjects are asked to do something they would not normally do or have to contribute a great deal of time or effort. Usually these rewards are small: a gift token or a small payment. Larger rewards might be seen as attracting volunteers who would not otherwise wish to take part in research, introducing undesired bias into the project.

# DATA COLLECTION

Once the research project is under way, data collection can begin. At the most basic level, data is either **quantitative** or **qualitative**. In health and social care research this data can be collected from a large range of sources and can take many forms. The same data might be collected in a quantitative form in one study and a qualitative form in another, through closed questions in a questionnaire or by interview, for example. The collection of some types of data may involve a degree of physical or psychological discomfort for the participants or subjects: for example, the collection of blood samples or interviews about being the victim of a crime. If this data is crucial to the project ethical approval can still be granted, but the researchers should always explore ways of collecting data that create less stress for the subjects or participants. Common types of data in health and social care research include:

- biochemical data – such as measurements of chemicals in blood or urine;
- physiological data – such as recordings of blood pressure or pulse;
- psychological data – levels of stress or anxiety;
- sociological data – information about lifestyle, hobbies, family structures.

# DATA COLLECTION TOOLS

At an early stage in study design the research team will decide on the data to be collected. Decisions about data collection tools can then be made. The choice of data collection tools is crucial to the eventual **validity** and **reliability** of the study. Reliability refers to the extent to which data collection methods will collect the same data on repeated occasions. The more consistently this occurs the more reliable the methods are. Validity refers to the extent to which data collection and analysis accurately measures what the researchers intend to measure. For example, recording the time a person takes to run a kilometre is a more valid way of measuring that person's fitness than simply asking: 'How long does it take you to run a kilometre?' Recording the time using a sensitive digital timing device will be a more reliable way of measuring the time than using the second hand of a watch.

Tools need to be as simple as possible, whether they are to be used by researchers or participants. They must be unambiguous, clear, consistent and unbiased. They do not always have to be created for an individual study. In fact there are many advantages in using data collection tools that have been developed and used by other researchers. These tools are likely to be valid and reliable, ensuring that they are acceptable ways of collecting particular data, so using them means that we do not have to design and test new tools before we embark on our study. Using established and recognised data collection tools also makes it easier for our results to be compared to those of other studies now and in the future. Here are some examples to choose from.

- *Checklists and proformas* – used to record pre-determined data, especially quantitative data.
- *Questionnaires* – used to record responses to pre-set questions. These questions can be closed (allowing only 'Yes/No' responses), restricted (offering a range of responses, such as 'Yes', 'No' and 'Don't know') or open (inviting the respondent to write about their thoughts, suggestions or criticisms). They can be self-completed by the respondent or they can be used by the researcher during a structured interview.
- *Diaries* – either completed by research participants or, in some research methodologies, by the researcher.
- *Audio or videotapes* – used to record interviews or other events.
- *Interviews* – these can be structured, semi-structured or unstructured (see below).
- *Artefacts* – objects or pieces of equipment relating to the subject of the research. These may be pre-existing or they may be produced by participants (for example, drawings or other artworks, stories, photographs).

In health and social care research data collection is often undertaken by the use of interviews or observation. Qualitative designs are normally associated with these methods, although quantitative data can also be collected using these methods. Each one is worth further consideration here.

## Interviews

Interviews can usually be described as structured, semi-structured or unstructured depending on how tightly the interview process is controlled within the study.

Structured interviews are tightly controlled. Each interview carried out in the study uses the same questions, often using exactly the same words to ask them, asking them in the same order each time. This creates a high level of consistency between each interview, but does not allow the interview to deal with issues of importance to the participant that have not been 'built in' to the pre-arranged questions.

Unstructured interviews start with a general statement or question, such as: 'Please tell me about your experience of being unemployed'. After this the interview can cover any subject or topic that the interviewee wishes to raise. This gives the interviewee a high level of control and means that each interview can be very different from the others. This approach is popular with **phenomenological** researchers, but can create a vast amount of data which is time-consuming to classify and interpret.

Semi-structured interviews are perhaps the commonest form to be found in health and social care research. They combine the control over design found in the structured approach with the freedom for the participant offered by the unstructured approach.

## Observation

A key characteristic of observational research is the level of participation in the situation on the part of the researcher. In a participant observational study the researcher takes an active role in the situation being studied. In a non-participant observation the researcher does nothing more than observe the situation, taking no part in the actions being studied.

In practice, most observers in health and social care research are present in the situation being studied but the level of involvement they have varies tremendously. Observers need to be clear about their roles before beginning a period of observation, to ensure consistency in every setting on each occasion. They also need to be clear about the extent to which they will maintain their roles in exceptional circumstances, when doing so may be unethical or dangerous.

### Key Question 3 – Problems in observational studies

If you were the researcher in the following situations, would you maintain your role?

- You are a non-participant observer, studying care in a residential home. The research requires that you do not interact with residents or carers, but that you simply watch and record certain activities. One morning you see two carers verbally abusing a resident for a few seconds.
- You are a non-participant observer, studying the activities of a community mental health team. You can engage in general conversation with clients and workers, but you should not discuss or participate in care activities. During a home visit a client falls and hits his head, becoming unconscious. The mental health worker asks you to call an ambulance while she begins to give first aid.
- You are acting as a researcher in a project studying fundraising work in a large charity. You are an active participant observer, fully immersed in the fundraising work. After a few weeks one fundraiser tells you of a scheme which enables each fundraiser to divert £50 each week to their personal bank account. 'Everyone does it and the charity won't miss it.'

## ISSUES IN DATA COLLECTION

Data collection is fraught with problems of reliability and validity. Can we, as potential users of research evidence, be sure that data was collected accurately, consistently and honestly? Probably not, but we trust that this is what happened. Unfortunately our trust can sometimes be misplaced as data is not always collected as reliably as we might hope.

## Blinding

It is possible to reduce bias and improve reliability in a study by **blinding** participants or researchers to some aspect of the research process. This ensures that a key piece of information is not known and therefore does not impact on the way in which the researcher or participant acts. Studies can be **double-blind** or **single-blind**.

In a double-blind study both researcher and participant are blinded. In a single-blind study either the researcher or participant will be blinded. In an unblinded study neither the researcher nor the participant is blinded. Drug trials are double-blinded whenever possible and this is usually a relatively simple process. Subjects are allocated to an **intervention group** or **control group**, but are not told to which group they have actually been allocated. Researchers collect and analyse data but do not know the group to which the person the data refers to was allocated. If it is possible to blind either the researcher or the participant but not both then the study is a single-blind one. This can occur in research into socially-complex health or social care interventions. For example, a study of a new mobility aid for people with arthritis might test its effectiveness by comparing a group of people using the aid with a group of people who do not use the aid. It would be possible to organise data collection and analysis so that the researcher was blinded to each individual's group allocation, but the participants would clearly know if they were using the aid.

## Hawthorne Effect

Imagine for a moment that you are doing something you enjoy and feel confident about, such as driving a car, cooking a meal or playing a computer game. Then imagine that a famous expert in that activity arrives, tells you that they will be watching you very closely and declares that they will give you an assessment of your ability at the end of the day. Do you still feel confident? Do you carry on exactly as before? Or do you get nervous, fumble and make simple mistakes?

Knowing that you are in a research project can affect your behaviour. Having a researcher observing you can affect your actions to an even greater extent. The impact that a researcher can have on the situation being observed is known as the Hawthorne Effect.

The Hawthorne Effect was originally identified during experiments at the Hawthorne factory of the Western Electric Company in Chicago in the late 1920s and early 1930s (Diaper, 1990). Since then most health and social care researchers appear to have become familiar with the idea, even if few of us have read the original papers. It's an important effect to consider in any project where individuals know they are being studied, because it may well introduce a bias into the data being collected and so create invalid and unreliable results.

If the Hawthorne Effect was consistent then it would be easy to deal with. Unfortunately, it isn't consistent and is affected by different variables in each research project. Indeed, there may be more than one 'Hawthorne Effect' and it is impossible to measure accurately the extent of the effect when designing a study (Holden, 2001). Even though it cannot be measured accurately you should always consider a study's potential Hawthorne Effect when you read a report of its findings.

## CONFIDENTIALITY AND ANONYMITY

Data collection should always be carried out in ways that ensure confidentiality and anonymity. The two concepts are related, but focus on different aspects of research. Confidentiality refers to the ways in which raw data is collected and stored. Anonymity refers to the identity of the data supplier: the participant.

When researchers collect data and store it prior to analysis they must ensure that both these processes are confidential. Participants who have provided data, especially through recorded interviews or observations, must feel confident that this data will be seen by only the research team involved in the study. It must be clear, for example, that their managers, their health or social care workers or their colleagues will not have access to this data.

After analysis, some data will be included in the research report and so it is no longer confidential. Data can, however, be kept anonymous. At the earliest possible stage of data collection and analysis the researchers should ensure that data is coded or classified in such a way that it cannot be traced back to an identifiable individual by anyone other than the researchers themselves. Data that is used in the final report must not be attributable to an identifiable individual either. The anonymising of data is relatively easy in studies that use large sample sizes and collect **quantitative data**, for example responses to closed questions in surveys or biochemical data such as blood glucose measurements. Small-scale studies collecting data from interviews, audio recordings or diaries must ensure that the raw data sources, such as the diaries or the interview recordings, are securely stored. Individual participants must be referred to using pseudonyms or codes in any report of the study that is made public.

## SUMMARY

Although many researchers see data analysis as the most important stage of the research process, reliable analysis can occur only if the data is itself reliable. Recruitment and data collection are critical stages in the creation of a body of data. Effective recruitment needs a thorough knowledge of the total population of interest, including the key characteristics of the population on which selection criteria will be based. Whether the study sample is selected randomly or purposively the steps of the activity need to be well-planned and should be reported clearly.

The reasons behind the chosen collection strategies should also be well thought out. Data collection choices impact on the analysis and discussion as they directly influence the nature of the data that the researcher obtains. Prospective users of research findings need to understand not only what information the data can give them but also what it cannot.

---

### KEY LEARNING POINTS

- Recruitment to a study should be based on clear criteria which define the population of interest and the conditions that an individual must meet in order to be suitable for selection.
- Randomised sampling aims to create a study sample which is representative of the population of interest.
- Purposive sampling is used to select a sample that has specific characteristics but is not necessarily representative.
- Data collection tools should be selected to ensure that the required data is obtained in a consistent and accurate fashion.
- Study participants must be assured of confidentiality and anonymity before they commit to taking part in a study.

---

# FURTHER READING

Department of Health (2005) *Research governance framework for health and social care*. London: Department of Health

Fox, M, Martin, P and Green, G (2007) *Doing practitioner research*. London: Sage

Malterud, K (2001) 'Qualitative research: standards, challenges, and guidelines'. *The Lancet*, 358: 483–8

National Health and Medical Research Council of Australia (1999) *National statement on ethical conduct in research involving humans*. **www.nhmrc.gov.au/publications/synopses/_files/e35.pdf** (6 March 2007)

Parahoo, K (2006) *Nursing research: principles, process and issues* (2nd edn). London: Palgrave Macmillan

Yin, RK (2003) *Case study research design and methods. Applied social research methods series. Volume 5*. Thousand Oaks: Sage

# Chapter 6

# Data Analysis

This chapter discusses the following topics.

- Major ways of analysing data – their benefits and drawbacks.

- Quantitative and qualitative.

- Levels of quantitative data analysis.

- Major statistical tests.

- Types of qualitative analysis.

- Major methods of qualitative analysis.

## INTRODUCTION

Data that has not been analysed can give us some information, but it's only after analysis that the researchers will feel confident in reaching conclusions and making recommendations that might be of use for health and social care practice. Analysis is the stage in the research process where sense is made of the data, turning what can seem to be a meaningless collection of numbers or words into a body of evidence upon which practitioners or policy-makers may base major decisions.

Data analysis is not, of course, a straightforward process. Once again we will be discussing a wide range of classifications, debates, arguments and methods, even though the basic division is a simple one. Analysis is qualitative or quantitative, but each of these two approaches has a wide choice of more specific methods and this choice seems to be increasing every year.

# QUANTITATIVE ANALYSIS AND QUALITATIVE ANALYSIS: THE SAME BUT DIFFERENT?

Before we look at quantitative and qualitative analysis separately I want to look at them together, to consider their similarities before we look at their differences. All data analysis attempts to do the same thing: to make sense of data that has been collected, in order to provide us with information. Analysis involves 'examining, categorizing, tabulating, testing or otherwise recombining' evidence (Yin, 2003, p.109). The information that results from these processes might be used to explain past events, establish relationships or develop understanding of experiences. Some analysis will be incredibly successful, some will fail miserably. Some will enable practitioners to make major improvements in treatment or care, some will mislead us. It doesn't matter if the analysis is quantitative or qualitative.

There are other similarities, which have been summarised by Onwuegbuzie and Leech (2005). Analysis attempts to answer a research question through constructing explanations and speculating about the reasons why outcomes arise. It involves extracting meaning from data. It involves the reduction of data, making it less complicated and more understandable. In health and social care it is an attempt to understand human behaviour. Once again, it doesn't matter if it's quantitative or qualitative. Of course, not everyone agrees with this perspective. Lincoln and Guba (1985, p.333), two leading supporters of naturalistic research, emphasise that qualitative analysis is about the reconstruction of raw data into 'meaningful wholes' and so is not about reduction but about induction.

So why do so many research textbooks, including this one, separate qualitative and quantitative analysis? I think there are two main reasons. First, because although quantitative and qualitative analysis share the same aims and intentions, they use different methods and deal with raw material presented in different forms. When you are trying to help students make sense of analysis, or when you are a student trying to develop your own understanding of the process, there is a certain logic to separating the methods in this way. All the methods that use numbers, statistics and mathematics fit neatly into one broad category. All the methods that work with text or words fit neatly into another category. After all, a modern secondary school education prepares your mind in this way by teaching separate maths and English lessons.

The second reason is specific to the development of health and social care research. It's what writers such as Onwuegbuzie and Leech (2005) refer to as the Paradigm Wars. The concept of Paradigm Wars overdramatises the disagreements between the more extreme supporters of the two opposing **paradigms** of positivism and interpretivism. It implies clear distinctions not only between the paradigms but also at the levels of methodology and methods. Onwuegbuzie and Leech (2005, p.217) refer to two research 'subcultures': the 'positivistic quantitative' subculture and the 'interpretivist qualitative' subculture. This notion of subcultures suggests two distinct and opposing camps of researchers: a positivist camp where only experimental methodologies and quantitative methods are allowed, and an interpretivist camp which uses only naturalistic methodologies and qualitative methods. It's true that some researchers will stick doggedly to a very narrow idea of what constitutes 'research', but increasing numbers are taking a more flexible position. Even those researchers who carry out only experimental studies using quantitative data analysis will recognise the relevance and **validity** of naturalistic designs, and vice versa.

As I hope I have made clear in earlier chapters, I think that health and social care research is now too flexible to sustain such Paradigm Wars. But we still think of methods of data analysis as sitting in one or other camp, because the distinction between the analysis of numbers and analysis of words is such an easy one to recognise. Data collection methods such as surveys, interviews or observation can be used to collect **quantitative** and **qualitative data**. Data analysis methods are designed for text or numbers. If you have a very rigid and inflexible approach to research then it is easy to link one set of data analysis methods with one particular paradigm. You can perpetuate the Paradigm Wars, but I can think of little benefit in doing so.

I will now go on to discuss quantitative and qualitative methods of data analysis separately. But remember, data analysis in health and social care research is characterised more by similarities than by differences.

## QUANTITATIVE ANALYSIS

Quantitative analysis attempts to make sense of numbers. But, as Parahoo (1997, p.339) notes, 'numbers in themselves have no intrinsic worth: they have to be given meaning by those who use them'. Much of this giving of meaning has to come before the data collection stage of a study. For example, if my project will collect data about urine output I need to decide what units of measurement I will use: a measurement of 100 millilitres is very different from a measurement of 100 fluid ounces. In a study of people's ideas about the quality of care in a day centre, if I ask each person to score the care on a scale of 1 to 10 then I need to make it clear that 1 represents the best care and 10 the worst to avoid confusing the participants.

If I don't clearly define what numbers mean before I start collecting data then my data will be meaningless and my analysis will be unreliable. As long as I collect reliable data my analysis has the potential to provide meaningful information. In quantitative analysis there are two basic forms in which this information can be provided: levels of measurement and statistical analysis.

# MEASUREMENT SCALES

We often use quantitative data to measure things, so that we can understand those things more clearly. Some of our measurements in day-to-day life are quite subjective and lack the ability to be interpreted reliably and consistently. Applying numerical values to these measures helps to achieve **reliability** and consistency.

If we say that someone is 'tall', or that the weather is 'cold', or that a new pair of shoes is 'expensive' we are making judgements about height, temperature or cost. But our judgements might not be shared, or understood in the same way, by others. If we say instead that someone is 180 cms in height, or that the temperature is 6 °C, or that the shoes cost £200, we are applying more accurate and objective measurements. Assuming that our information is correct, no-one will argue with our measurements. A 198 cm tall millionaire from Alaska might, of course, argue that 180 cms is not tall, 6 °C is not cold and £200 is not expensive, but this is a disagreement about *interpretation* of measurement, not about the measurement itself.

Presenting our data in numerical form enables us to compare data. The levels of comparison that can be made vary according to the types of measurement that we can achieve. Statisticians generally refer to four measurement scales, each one providing a more complex level of information than the one preceding it. The four scales are:

1 nominal;
2 ordinal;
3 interval;
4 ratio.

Nominal scales allow us to allocate individual subjects or outcomes to different categories. Stating that subject A is female and subject B is male allows us to allocate each person to a distinct group, female or male. But we can't go on to make any quantitative judgements: we can't say that subject A has more 'femaleness' than subject B has 'maleness'.

Ordinal scales take us one stage further, enabling us to place subjects in some sort of order. An example of an ordinal scale might be judgements about the depth of colour of subjects' hair. We can say that subjects A, B and C all have brown hair, but that C's is darker than B's and A's is darker than C's. An ordinal scale does not, however, enable us to quantify the degree of difference. We can't say that C's hair is 11% darker than B's and A's is 16% darker than C's.

Another ordinal scale is the type used to measure a person's satisfaction with something: a patient's or client's satisfaction with care, for example (Cornish, 1998). A satisfaction survey might ask patients to rank their care as 'excellent', 'good', 'average', 'poor', or 'very poor'. It's easy to see that 'good' is better than 'average' but we can't tell by how much it's better. Nor can we tell if a rating of good was almost an excellent rating or only just better than an average rating.

Interval scales enable us to identify differences with greater accuracy than ordinal scales. They offer us equal distances between values and allow us to place those values on a continuum. One of the best examples of an interval scale is the Centigrade scale for temperature measurement. This scale enables us to use specific values with constant, regular, differences between these values. So we know that the difference between 10 °C and 11 °C is the same as the difference between 31 °C and 32 °C. Interval scales don't have absolute zero points however, so we can't say that 20 °C is twice as warm as 10 °C, because temperatures can fall below 0 °C.

Scales with an absolute zero point as well as equal intervals between values and a clear continuum of values are known as ratio scales. Height measurement is a practical example of a ratio scale. The difference between 5 cm and 10 cm is the same as that between 95 cm and 100 cm. A height of 165 cm is taller than one of 162 cm. More importantly, there is a real zero point: 0 cm equals no height. This means that we can state relationships between two measurements more precisely. A person who is 200 cm tall *is* twice the height of one who is 100 cm tall.

Each of these scales allows us to present data in numerical form. A nominal scale where people are categorised as 'male' or 'female' allows the researcher to allocate a number to each category: 0 for male and 1 for female, for example. The researcher can allocate a number to each category in an ordinal scale just as easily, so that 'excellent' equals 5 and 'very poor' equals 1. Interval and ratio scales tend to have numerical values already.

This level of quantitative information is useful in itself, but rather limited. It tells us something about each individual subject or participant in a study, but not about the participants as a group, nor about an individual participant's place within the group. To be able to reach conclusions about relationships the researcher needs to carry out some statistical analysis at a more complex level.

## TYPES OF STATISTICAL ANALYSIS

In this discussion I will divide statistical analysis into two types: **descriptive** and **inferential statistics**. This is the most basic division you can find in the research literature and it is used by authors such as Parahoo (1997). Other authors use different classifications, based on alternative ways of defining categories. Mathers and Huang (1998) refer to **parametric** and **non-parametric** statistics, based on the types of data they are used to make sense of. Clifford (1997) subdivides inferential statistics into two categories, inferential and correlational.

## Descriptive statistics

Descriptive statistics provide us with information about the data as a whole. They summarise this data and enable the reader to gain a clear idea about the body of results in terms of their similarities and differences. Descriptive statistics normally provide information about three areas: frequency, central tendency and dispersion (Parahoo, 1997).

### *Frequency*

Frequency is usually reported as absolute numbers, proportions or percentages. Each way of reporting tells us how many of the sample share a particular characteristic, response or viewpoint. Let's take a research study of 100 social workers as an example. If the researchers want to report the number of male and female social workers they can do so by telling us the numbers of each, say 60 women and 40 men. They could also express these numbers as fractions of the total sample, giving proportions of $^3/_5$ women and $^2/_5$ men. They could also provide us with the information in percentages: 60% women and 40% men. In this example each approach works equally well, but once the numbers become more complicated proportions or percentages can offer a clearer and more consistent approach than the use of absolute numbers.

Let's assume that the researchers asked the social workers to agree or disagree with the statement that 'social workers should retire on their 50th birthdays' and that 48 female respondents and 32 male respondents agreed while 12 female and 8 male respondents disagreed. The absolute numbers tell us that more women than men agreed. This is true, but we need to remember that more women than men were asked to respond. Using fractions we can see that $^4/_5$ of women and $^4/_5$ of men agreed. Using percentages we can see that 80% of each group agreed. In other words, the frequency of agreement was the same in both groups.

### *Central tendency*

Measures of central tendency tell us about common features of a set of data, particularly about the midpoints of the range of responses. The commonest measure of central tendency is the mean. The median and the mode can also be calculated relatively easily but are not usually as useful.

A set of ten responses will help to illustrate the three measures of central tendency. Let's assume that they are scores out of ten given by respondents when asked to rate the quality of service provided by a housing association:

4, 4, 5, 6, 6, 6, 7, 7, 8, 8.

The mean, or arithmetic average, is calculated by adding up the scores and dividing the result by the number of individual scores. In this case we get 61 divided by 10, so the mean is 6.1.

The median is the point which 'divides the distribution of scores into two equal halves' (Cornish, 1998, p.8). With an odd number of responses the median is the middle score. With an even number take the scores either side of the midpoint, add them together and divide by 2. In our example the median is (6+6)÷2, which equals 6.

The mode is the most frequently occurring response. In this example it is also 6.

All three measures in this example are close together: 6.1, 6 and 6. This is not always the case.

Let's assume that the ten responses gave the following scores:

1, 2, 3, 4, 7, 8, 9, 9, 9, 9.

With these scores the mean is still 6.1. The median is now 7.5. The mode becomes 9.

I hope you can see from these two basic examples that measures of central tendency don't on their own offer us a clear description of a set of data. We need to know about the variation in data as well as similarities.

## Key Question 1: Mean, median and mode

In an 'out of hours' care centre the following numbers of people were seen each hour from 0800 to 2200 on a Sunday:

6, 6, 10, 8, 13, 10, 6, 7, 20, 14, 11, 6, 12, 4, 2.

- What was the mean attendance per hour?
- What figure represents the median attendance?
- What number is the mode attendance?

- What does the data tell you about the centre's activity?
- What conclusions, if any, can you draw from these figures?

## Measures of dispersion

Measures of dispersion or variability (Cornish, 1998) help us to understand the ways in which data are spread or dispersed. Three commonly used measures of dispersion are the range, distribution and standard deviation.

The range is a reasonably simple measure. It refers to the gap between the highest and lowest values in a sequence. In our first example (page 78) the range is 4–8: in our second it's 1–9.

Distribution refers to the way in which data is spread, or distributed, around the mean value. A normal distribution occurs when values are spread reasonably equally above and below the mean, giving a curve that resembles a bell when values are plotted on a graph. Distributions can also be abnormal, skewed to the left or to the right of the graph.

Standard deviation (SD) gives us further information about the distribution of data. Specifically, this measurement tells us about the extent to which scores are spread around the mean. A small SD suggests that the values are clustered around the mean, a large SD suggests that they are spread more widely (Cornish, 1998). A single SD either side of the mean will include about 68% of the data: two SDs either side of the mean will include 95% of the data: three SDs either side will include almost all of the data.

Our two sets of test results can help me to illustrate this.

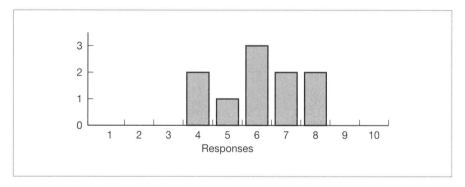

**Figure 1**

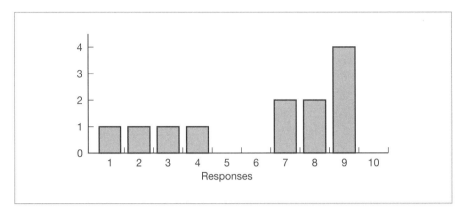

**Figure 2**

In Figure 1 the data has a mean of 6.1 and a median of 6. You can see that the distribution is roughly symmetrical: that is, equal numbers of responses fall on either side of the mean and median. The graph shows a 'bell-shaped' appearance, indicating a normal distribution.

In Figure 2 the mean is still 6.1 but the median is 7.5. There were no scores of 5 or 6 in the data. The distribution is skewed and abnormal.

## Inferential statistics

Few research projects are able to study an entire population of interest and so researchers must study samples of varying size. If they then wish to show that findings within the sample are generalisable to the population as a whole they need to provide evidence in support of their claim. Inferential statistics can provide this evidence: they allow us to *infer* that findings will apply to the whole population, not just to the sample.

A quick check of textbooks and websites will easily find at least ten or twelve inferential statistical tests that are routinely used in health and social care research. These tests are usually classified as **parametric** or **non-parametric**, to distinguish the level of measurement that needs to be possible in order for a test to be used.

Parametric tests can be used only when interval or ratio level measures exist and when data are normally distributed. Non-parametric tests can be applied to nominal or ordinal level data and do not need a normal distribution. Parametric tests are usually seen as more powerful than non-parametric ones.

Researchers cannot therefore simply choose any inferential statistical test, they must use one which matches the criteria for distribution and levels of measurement. Because of this, researchers can select the appropriate test by following a standard decision-making process, gradually eliminating tests until the appropriate choice remains.

## KEY CASE 1: Inferential statistics

The following are examples of different statistical tests that can be used to help researchers investigate relationships between sets of results.

Non-parametric tests.
- Chi-Square Test [written as chi2].
- Mann-Whitney U Test [U].
- Wilcoxon Signed Rank Test [W].
- Kruskal-Wallis Test [H].
Parametric tests.
- t-Test [t] – for related or unrelated data.
- Pearson Product Moment Correlation [r].
- Analysis of Variance [ANOVA: written as [F] – for related or unrelated data].

(All examples from Cornish, 1998)

## Calculating uncertainty

Although we have a tendency to use phrases such as 'research has shown', few health and social care researchers would claim that their results can be applied to the real world with 100% certainty. Instead they will carry out further calculations to estimate the degree of certainty that they can apply to the results of their studies. Two estimates of accuracy are commonly used in health and social care research: probability and **confidence intervals**.

Probability is usually shown by the $p$-value. In research this is used to indicate the likelihood that a result has occurred by chance, rather than because there is a genuine relationship between variables. If a result achieves a predetermined $p$-value, or less, then it is said to be statistically significant.

$P$-values are expressed as decimal numbers, so you will commonly see $p$-values of, for example, 0.05, or 0.01, or 0.001. Most researchers take a $p$-value of 0.05 or less as being statistically significant, although this is a fairly arbitrary figure (Coggon $et$ $al$, 1993).

A $p$-value of 0.05 is stating that the likelihood of a result occurring by chance is $^5/_{100}$ or 1 in 20: a $p$-value of 0.01 means that the likelihood is 1 in 100. The smaller the $p$-value, the more statistically significant a result is said to be.

The confidence interval seems to have become a standard measure of certainty in health and social care research in recent years. A confidence interval is 'a range within which, assuming there are no biases in the study method, the true value for the population parameter might be expected to lie' (Coggan *et al* 1993, p.62). Usually it is expressed as a 95% confidence interval [95% CI], as an additional note of caution. In other words, the research team is stating that they are confident that in 95% of cases (that is, 19 out of 20) the true result in the population as a whole will be somewhere within the range of values stated.

Let's take a new example. A study of social care finds that in its sample of 100 people the average waiting time for referral to a specialist service was 16 days. The researchers will not simply state that 16 days would be the average waiting time in the population as a whole. They will calculate the range of values within which they predict the actual average is likely to fall, with 95% confidence. In the report they will state the study result and the likely true figure for the population as a whole in this way: 16 days, 95% CI:13–19 days. In other words, they are stating that in 19 out of 20 cases the average waiting time in the actual population will be somewhere between 13 and 19 days.

As a rule, small sample sizes will produce wider confidence intervals than large samples: that is, the bigger your sample the more certain you can be that your result is accurate.

## MAJOR METHODS OF QUALITATIVE ANALYSIS

Quantitative analysis may incorporate a wide range of analytical tests, but they are all essentially variations on a single theme: the creation of numerical data for analysis by statistical or mathematical means. Qualitative analysis, by comparison, draws on a more diverse range of strategies and is able to make use of raw data in a greater variety of forms.

Most qualitative research produces text. This can be created directly, through written responses to open survey questions, or diaries written by research participants. It can also be produced indirectly, through the transcribing of interview recordings. But qualitative analysis is not limited to the use of data in text form. It has also developed strategies for analysing other forms of data, such as artwork, architectural plans or objects such as surgical instruments.

We noted earlier that qualitative methods are characterised by a great deal of debate about which method is best, so you will not be surprised to hear that qualitative analysis cannot be neatly classified. Clifford (1997, p.133) takes the simplest view, stating that: 'However data are collected, the process of analysis in qualitative research designs is known as content analysis'. But this is an overly-simplistic, not to say incorrect, view of qualitative analysis.

There are well over 30 different forms of qualitative data analysis identified in the literature. Grbich (2007) offers a particularly detailed classification, identifying around 35 techniques which she groups together under broader methodological headings. These include:

- classical **ethnography** – frame analysis, social network analysis, event analysis;
- **grounded theory** – Straussian and Glaserian analytical approaches;
- feminist research – memory work;
- content analysis;
- narrative analysis – socio-linguistic, socio-cultural;
- conversation analysis;
- discourse analysis;
- visual interpretation – ethnographic, historical, structural and post-structural;
- semiotic analysis.

Miles and Huberman (1994) add at least four more:

- case analysis;
- cross-case analysis;
- comparative analysis;
- causal analysis.

It's difficult to tell if these types of analysis are all distinct from each other, or whether some of them represent small variations in approach or the same methods applied to different data sources. But it's clear that there are many ways of analysing data qualitatively. Thankfully, a small number of methods predominate in health and social care research and I want to discuss only two of them:

- thematic analysis;
- constant comparison.

## Thematic analysis

**Thematic analysis** is one of the 'most useful and most widely used' methods of qualitative data analysis (Grbich 2007, p.36). In a thematic approach analysis takes place once all the data has been collected. It is, according to Grbich (2007, p.16) 'a process of segmentation, categorisation and relinking of aspects of the database prior to the final interpretation.' It is advocated by Holliday (2007, p.94), who describes it as an approach in which 'all the data is taken holistically and rearranged under themes which emerge as running through its totality'. It is also the method of qualitative analysis which I use in my own work, partly because I find it to be fairly straightforward and partly because it is less likely to be shrouded in the almost impenetrable jargon which makes many other techniques extremely difficult to understand.

In thematic analysis the researcher reduces the data into groups which are meaningful and relevant to the subject. Words or phrases in the text can be identified and coded. Codings eventually lead to the identification of themes or groups that can be organised and classified. The data is allocated to these groups, which enable interpretation of the data and therefore description or explanation of the phenomenon being studied.

## KEY CASE 2: A study of e-learning in the education of student nurses

In a recent study of an international e-learning project called a 'Community of Practice' (Lindsay, 2007) I invited participants to evaluate the project design and implementation. Eleven participants out of the total of 15 took part in the evaluation: a response rate of 73%. In response to three open questions about the project the respondents made 31 separate comments. Through thematic analysis and coding I eventually identified three themes which enabled me to classify the data: concept, content and implementation. Two of these themes, content and implementation, each included three smaller subthemes.

These themes and subthemes developed from the data: in other words, they are the result of my (hopefully unbiased) interpretation of participants' responses.

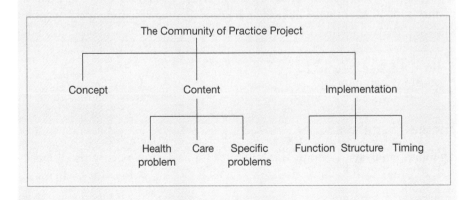

## Constant comparison

This method of data analysis was developed by Glaser and Strauss in the 1960s as part of their development of **grounded theory**, which we discussed in Chapter 3. Lincoln and Guba (1985) note that Glaser and Strauss intended constant comparison to be a way of deriving or grounding their theory development, not just as a way of analysing data, but in health and social care research it is more commonly used as a means of data analysis. Interestingly, Lincoln and Guba also note that Glaser and Strauss saw their approach as part of a positivist paradigm, even though constant comparison is now firmly rooted in naturalistic methodologies.

Constant comparison is similar to thematic analysis, in that the researcher reviews and interrogates the data in order to produce a meaningful, organised, classification. However, a key difference is in the way that the process is undertaken, or more specifically in the relationship between data collection and analysis. In constant comparison the researcher begins to analyse the data as soon as it begins to emerge, rather than at the end of the data collection process. Early data analysis informs data collection and can lead to developments in the collection process. For example, early analysis might lead to a revision of the interview schedule, or a deliberate move towards the selection of participants who can best assist in testing out early ideas.

### Key Question 2: Qualitative data analysis

Select a database of your choice (for example, Medline or Google Scholar) and search for research publications which use three different types of qualitative data analysis, one from each of the lists on page 83. For example, search for 'thematic analysis', 'discourse analysis' and 'case analysis'. Identify papers that use these types of analysis and then read them.

- How do they present their analysis and findings?
- How does this vary between the types of analysis?
- How does this compare to the ways in which other papers analyse and present quantitative data?

## SUMMARY

As a reader and potential user of research and research findings you do not have to analyse data yourself. However, having at least some understanding of the process means that you can make judgements about the quality of data analysis and do not simply have to accept that it is valid and reliable. This understanding is invaluable because, as I have already said, just because a research report has been published doesn't mean that it is necessarily of good quality.

---

## KEY LEARNING POINTS

- Data can be analysed quantitatively or qualitatively.
- These two approaches to analysis have many similarities as well as differences.
- There is no single, universally applicable, approach to quantitative or qualitative data analysis: researchers should select the best approach for their data.
- Different ways of analysing data produce different results: always consider what the analysis of data might fail to tell you, as well as what it does tell you.

---

## FURTHER READING

These texts all focus on either quantitative or qualitative analysis, offering a much more in-depth discussion of analysis than this book contains.

Coggon, D, Rose, G and Barker, DJP (1993) *Epidemiology for the uninitiated* (3rd edn). London: BMJ Publishing Group. This is a brief book, focusing on the use of statistical analysis in the study of patterns of disease but offering plenty of information of use by health or social care practitioners.

Cornish, K (1998) *Trent focus for research and development in primary health care: An introduction to using statistics in research*. Nottingham: Trent Focus. This text and the one by Wharrad are both short papers targeted at beginning researchers. They are easy to read and concentrate on common approaches.

Grbich, C (2007) *Qualitative data analysis. An introduction*. London: Sage

Holliday, A (2007) *Doing and writing qualitative research* (2nd edn). London: Sage

Maltby, J, Day, L and Williams, G (2007) *Introduction to statistics for nurses*. Harlow: Pearson Education. This text provides a far more in-depth discussion of statistics than most nurses or health professionals will ever need. Its discussion of the use of software in data analysis is particularly useful.

Wharrad, H (1998) *Trent focus for research and development in primary health care: an introduction to experimental designs*. Nottingham: Trent Focus

# Chapter 7

# What do we Know Now? Communicating Research Findings

This chapter discusses the following topics.

- What can research tell us?

- Limits to research accuracy

- How do researchers tell us about their work?

## INTRODUCTION

We have spent much of the first part of this book discussing the production of research evidence so that you are able to make sense of findings that you read about in reports. There is one more stage of the research process to discuss in this way: the dissemination of research.

As a health and social care student or practitioner you may not see an understanding of the dissemination or communication process as crucial. But this process means that the information you receive is produced and distributed in ways that can, at best, help you to achieve a real insight into a research project or, at worst, can leave you confused and puzzled about the study, its results and its relevance to your work.

## WHAT CAN RESEARCH TELL US?

Health and social care students and professionals can show surprising faith in research findings. I often read assignments that refer to research findings with little or no attempt to critique them, treating the findings as both accurate and applicable to practice without bothering to assess this apparent accuracy and applicability. Professionals routinely seem happy to change practice on the basis of the findings of a single research project. Perhaps the commonest indicator of this faith is the use of the phrase 'research has shown'.

It's a phrase that health and social care lecturers, students and practitioners use regularly and which creates little, if any, comment, yet its use suggests a profound relationship between research and practice. 'Research has shown' suggests that the speaker or writer believes that research provides proof; that the results of a research project can offer us clear direction about our practice, its management and its delivery. But health and social care research rarely, if ever, offers us absolute proof that is universally applicable: research doesn't 'show'.

This is not to say that research is irrelevant, just that potential users must be clear about the extent to which they can use research findings. If you want to do this accurately then you need to be able to evaluate research findings and understand how researchers disseminate their findings.

As a health and social care researcher I am always conscious of the uses to which my research findings might be put. Partly, this is because I like to think that my research findings *will* be used. Partly, it's because I'm aware that my research findings are never 100% accurate and I am worried that someone may treat them as totally accurate and use them inappropriately. I'm not unusual in this: researchers from all paradigms will take great pains to ensure that their uncertainties are communicated clearly. We use **confidence intervals**, or measures of significance, or sections headed 'Limitations of the Study' to declare these uncertainties to our readers.

But if health and social care research doesn't show us proof, what does it offer to practitioners? The answer is: quite a lot. Each research study, as long as it's valid and reliable, tells us a little more about the world. Each project adds to our body of knowledge about health and social care and helps us to understand it better.

Because research is about understanding, it doesn't always have to tell us that a new thing is better than an old thing. There is a tendency in health and social care literature to look for projects that give 'positive' results. In other words, a study comparing a new drug with an old drug is of interest if it tells us that the new drug is a significant improvement, while a study of a new social work practice will be of interest if it suggests that this new practice offers better care than previous practices have done. This tendency is part of publication bias and, it has been suggested, it means that studies reporting negative or neutral results are less likely to get published. But as practitioners we should always look for studies with negative or neutral results, because they can be equally important for practice.

Negative results suggest that the new intervention being studied is less effective than previous practices. Neutral results suggest that a new intervention is no different in its effectiveness to older ones. Change is not always necessary or beneficial in health and social care and while negative or neutral results are less attractive to the media they are vital for practitioners to ensure that we do not adopt new drugs, strategies or practices for the sake of it. So health and social care research can:

- provide evidence in support of, or in opposition to, an existing theory or procedure;
- suggest the likely outcome of a course of action;
- support the development of a new policy or procedure;
- describe a situation;
- predict likely future events with a variable degree of accuracy.

Even if it rarely provides 100%, irrefutable, predictive and incontestable proof.

Researchers themselves usually recognise this. Quantitative analysis will include calculations of significance and calculations of accuracy, such as confidence intervals. Qualitative analysis does not offer us such mathematical measurements but its discussion should attempt to evaluate its levels of truthfulness or transferability, both of which are in their own ways attempts to define the accuracy of the findings.

Of course, many **interpretive** researchers might claim that their work should not be measured in terms of 'accuracy' because it is seeking to explain or simply describe a particular set of unique events from a specific viewpoint or perspective. It is not seeking to predict future events. But most health and social care practitioners want research to do just that: to predict ways in which they should practise for maximum effectiveness. The accuracy of a description or explanation is therefore of critical importance if the research is to be of any use in helping to develop evidence-based practice.

## LIMITS TO RESEARCH ACCURACY

Research projects in health and social care fail to achieve 100% accuracy for three reasons: the quality of their design, the quality of their execution and the nature of their subject-matter. All three of these factors interlink, but I will discuss each of them separately, beginning with the subject-matter.

Health and social care research deals with people and people are generally difficult research subjects. Their behaviour is affected by innumerable different influences, their response to treatment or care is the result of a seemingly infinite set of variables and their willingness to take part in research projects can be influenced by apparently unimportant and unpredictable factors. Trying to predict or describe the future behaviour of a group of people by making judgements about the past behaviour of a different group of people is fraught with difficulties. But this is what health and social care research often attempts to do and to do with as high a degree of accuracy as possible.

> ## Key Question 1
>
> Think about some of your friends.
>
> - How are they today?
> - Could you have predicted with 100% accuracy what they did today based on what they did yesterday?
> - Can you predict exactly how they will behave tomorrow based on what they did today?
> - Think about a research study with a sample of 1000 social services clients.
> - How accurately do you expect this study to predict the behaviour of the population based on this sample?
> - Do you expect it to be more accurate than your predictions of your friends' behaviour, or less?

Designing research projects is problematic. Most health and social care projects are small and even the largest must usually sample its subjects or participants. Other design limitations put further constraints on projects. Most projects have time limits on them, and financial limits, and ethical constraints. There are legal restrictions and geographical restrictions and methodological restrictions. Project design is all too often a compromise between what a researcher wants to do and what can be done.

Once the project is under way there are problems of execution, that is, of carrying it out. These problems can arise for predictable reasons, such as a high dropout rate, or for unpredictable reasons, such as the resignation of a key member of the research team or a sudden change in government policy which ends the activity the project hopes to study. However well-designed the study was, a failure to carry it out as intended will have a negative impact on its **reliability** and **validity** and, ultimately, on its results.

## Researcher honesty

Researchers could just make everything up. Why bother going to all the trouble of recruitment, **randomisation**, data collection and analysis when you can simply invent your results? Throughout this book I have discussed various possible sources of **bias** in research and in Chapter 5 we looked at the honesty of research participants, so it is only right that we should also consider the possibility of deliberate dishonesty on the part of the researchers themselves.

Having raised the issue, I would like immediately to declare my firm belief that the vast majority of health and social care researchers are honest in their work. Partly this is because I think that health and social care professionals are honest individuals, partly it's because I feel that researchers generally have little to gain by falsifying some or all of their work and partly it's because the communication process contains a series of defences against dishonest research. But researcher honesty isn't universal, as Key Case 1 shows.

## KEY CASE 1: Falsifying reseach

In 2005 *The Lancet*, one of the world's most highly-respected medical journals, published a paper by Sudbø and colleagues from Norway and the United States which reported on the use of non-steroidal anti-inflammatory drugs (NSAIDs) and oral cancer (Sudbø *et al*, 2005). The study concluded that NSAIDs were associated with a reduced risk of oral cancer.

In its issue of 21 January 2006 the journal reported its concern regarding the study, noting that newspapers were reporting not simply that the results were inaccurate but that Dr Sudbø had fabricated every piece of data (Horton, 2006a). In early February the journal retracted the article completely, noting that an investigation had found that the entire data set was fabricated (Horton, 2006b). A report in the *Guardian* newspaper stated that Dr Sudbø had invented all of the 908 patients in the study and had given 250 of them the same date of birth (Fouché, 2006). Dr Sudbø's entire body of research was scrutinised by an independent committee and was found to contain serious errors and fabrications.

## BUILDING A BODY OF RESEARCH

Accepting that individual research projects are seldom 100% accurate is crucial to your ability to appraise research effectively. Understanding the limitations of a study's design and execution enables you to have a much more realistic understanding of the research process and a clearer awareness of the uses of research findings for practitioners.

## Key Question 2

- How often is health and social care practice less than perfect?
- What gets in the way of achieving perfection?
- Does less-than-perfect practice still produce worthwhile results?
- What factors that affect practice may have an equal impact on research?

It is important to remember that we should not be basing health or social care practice on a single research project. Health and social care practitioners should be looking more widely, at a body of research which represents an accumulation of evidence from a range of projects. In almost every field of health and social care the body of research builds up over a period of time, with projects from different settings, using different methodologies and undertaken by researchers from different academic and professional backgrounds.

To use research findings effectively practitioners need to develop skills of analysis and critiquing. We also need to be able to search effectively, so that we can base our judgements on an understanding of the whole body of relevant research not just on the first two or three papers we find on the internet. We also need some understanding of why the research papers we read are available, and what process they have gone through before they achieve publication. This process is what I will now discuss.

## DISSEMINATING RESEARCH

When we talk about disseminating research, or research findings, we are talking about the various ways in which information about a research project can be made known. When you read a research paper you are taking part in this final stage of the research process. In fact, if no-one reads reports and articles, or listens to conference presentations, then a research project is not truly complete. Making your research findings known means that your work is open to scrutiny and criticism. It means that your design, analysis and conclusions can be studied, commented on and criticised by your fellow academics or practitioners. But it can also lead to your work being applauded as some of the best in its field, as ground-breaking, or as influencing major developments in practice or policy. As a researcher, dissemination creates the risk that your weaknesses will be exposed but it also offers the chance of international fame, even if this fame is limited to a small and specialised academic discipline.

You might think that when the time comes to write a report the hard work has been completed, but this isn't always the case. Dissemination isn't simply about making your research findings known, it's about making them known in the best possible way and about being prepared to defend them from criticism.

There are many ways to produce and make available a report of a research project, including:

• submitting your dissertation or thesis, if your research has been undertaken to gain a qualification;

- writing a report for, or presenting a seminar paper to, your colleagues and managers;
- writing a report for the organisation that funded your study;
- presenting a paper at a conference;
- publishing a paper in an academic or professional journal.

The last two are of particular importance to career researchers and academics and are worthy of further discussion.

## Conference presentation

Many researchers present their findings at conferences, before going on to publish papers about the study. Conferences are important events, enabling researchers to get together with others from their specialist fields in order to share ideas and keep up to date with the body of evidence. The growth of the internet, with its online journals and the ability to publish and read research reports easily and quickly, might be seen to render conferences obsolete, but this has not proved to be the case. Health and social care researchers enjoy meeting face-to-face and the networking activity that goes on at conferences is for many researchers even more important than the presentations themselves. Conference venues are also important. International conferences take place in some of the best known and most interesting places in the world and the attraction of conferences in places like Venice, Sydney or Vancouver should not be underestimated.

Conferences usually offer three ways for researchers to communicate formally about their work: the poster presentation, the parallel session and the keynote paper. Poster presentation is popular with junior or inexperienced researchers. Prior to the conference the researchers prepare a poster, often a laminated A1 sized sheet, containing important information about their study. The poster is then displayed at the conference, perhaps only for a single day. Often one of the poster's authors will be expected to stand by the poster during a lunch or tea break so that interested people can ask questions about the study.

Parallel sessions give researchers the chance to present their findings as short lectures of 15–20 minutes, followed by a question-and-answer session. As the name suggests, a number of sessions are held 'in parallel', with conference delegates choosing which one to attend. Research studies which are of interest to a minority of conference delegates have the opportunity to be presented in these sessions. Parallel sessions can be attended by large audiences, but they can also attract very small numbers: some years ago I was one of a panel of six researchers presenting to an audience of five delegates.

Posters and parallel sessions are usually selected competitively. Researchers submit brief abstracts outlining their poster or session to a 'scientific committee' which selects the submissions that best suit the conference, so a very popular conference may reject the majority of abstracts submitted. Keynote papers are different, as they are given by invited presenters and are often seen as major attractions for potential delegates. Keynote presenters at large international conferences are senior figures and can be leading researchers, academics or political figures.

## The publication process

Textbooks are not likely to be used to publish the first report of a research project, although research papers can be published in textbooks after they have appeared in journals. Most undergraduate research in health and social care, and a large amount of post-graduate research, never gets beyond the production of the dissertation or thesis. Many small, local, projects go no further than their local audiences. But for 'career researchers' the most desirable way of disseminating their work is by publishing, and by publishing in the most prestigious journal possible.

When you read a paper in an academic or professional journal you are almost certainly reading a paper that has already undergone critical appraisal before being published. Towards the end of a project, if not earlier, the research team will begin to think about the way in which they will make their work known.

Some projects will be written up in a single paper, summarising the entire project in 4000 or 5000 words. Other projects will be published in a series of papers, each focusing on a different aspect of the work and perhaps appearing in a series of different journals. The team will make a decision about which journal or journals they hope will publish their work, based on ideas about their intended audience, the ways in which they want to present their findings and the prestige of the journal. They will then contact their first-choice journal and ask if it would be interested in their work. If the answer is a positive one then the researchers will prepare their paper based on the journal's style guidelines. If the editors don't wish to consider the paper then the researchers will contact the next journal on their list, and so on. Manuscripts can be sent direct to an editor without asking if the journal would be interested, but if the paper is not of interest to the journal this can simply waste the researchers' time.

Once a journal receives the manuscript of the paper the editor will send it to two or three expert reviewers. This is usually a **double-blind** process: the authors do not know who is reviewing their paper, the reviewers don't know who wrote the paper. The reviewers should also not be aware of the identities of the other reviewers. This process resembles the way in which assignments are marked in college or university, so you might find it helpful to think of the reviewing process in that way.

The reviewers have three options. They can propose that a paper should be accepted for publication, that it should be rejected, or that it should be revised by the authors according to the reviewers' suggestions before being re-submitted. Highly prestigious or popular journals such as the *British Medical Journal* receive very high numbers of submissions and will reject most of them. Less popular journals receive far fewer submissions and are more likely to ask authors to revise their papers so that they can be reconsidered. Having your paper accepted without the need to make any changes is, in my experience at least, a fairly rare occurrence.

After this process of revision and re-appraisal is complete the paper will, hopefully, be accepted for publication and then it will finally appear in the journal. This process can take several months, so that the paper you read might well be based on a project that was completed over a year before publication. Many journals help you to know how long the process has taken by giving details of the dates when a paper was first submitted and when it was accepted. A well-written paper should also give information regarding the dates of data collection, which can be years before the date on which the paper was actually submitted. This gives the reader important information about the recency of the data and the likely relevance of the study to current practice.

I don't expect that many readers of this book will be publishing papers in the near future, but I would urge you to read a few sets of guidelines for authors as a way of understanding the publication process more clearly. Many of the students I teach about research are extremely critical of published research papers because they see them as lacking detail about the studies. They will tell me that a paper fails to include a copy of the questionnaire used in the study, or doesn't tell them enough about the researchers' qualifications or experience, or doesn't give enough examples of raw data, or interview transcripts. While all of these criticisms are usually true, they are not always fair, especially when the authors of the paper are blamed for these omissions.

Publication is tightly controlled by the publishing companies and authors are constrained by journal guidelines regarding what they can and can't include in their papers. Most journals have strict limits on the length of articles, on the use of graphs, tables or illustrations and on the way in which references are identified. Information is almost always left out of articles and in many cases what is left out is of more interest to practitioners or to new researchers than it is to experienced researchers and academics. Academic journals do not pay their authors and in some cases they may even charge authors for the inclusion of photographs or illustrations: unless your research grant includes the costs of the publication process few researchers will be willing to fund them from their own pockets.

> ## Key Question 3: Author guidelines
>
> Find the author guidelines for some of the best-known health and social care research journals. They are often on the inside front or back pages of the journal or can be found on the publisher's website.
>
> - What rules do they insist on?
> - How restrictive or helpful do you think they might be for an author?
>
> Think about how the finished article will be influenced by these guidelines.

## The internet and publication

The internet has opened up new opportunities for publication, in the form of internet-only journals such as the *Internet Journal of Allied Health Sciences and Practice*, or *Early Childhood Research and Practice*. It has also made research papers more readily accessible through databases, search engines and the creation of web versions of published papers that can be obtained via your personal computer.

Established health and social care journals have used the internet with varying degrees of success or imagination. Used effectively, the internet enables journals to offer 'pre-publication' versions of research papers or to expand the number of diagrams, tables or images that accompany an article. The *British Medical Journal* has developed a 'Rapid Response' facility where readers of a research paper can post their comments or criticisms on the journal's website within minutes of reading the article. This is a very useful resource for students as it enables you to see the ways in which experienced researchers and practitioners critique published research papers.

Conference papers can also be published on a conference website, greatly increasing their potential audience. Some conferences are now held on the internet, creating 'virtual' conferences and avoiding the need for participants to travel thousands of miles in order to attend.

The openness of the internet can cause problems. Anyone can set up a website, or contribute to a discussion forum, and can spread misinformation deliberately or accidentally. Whenever you access evidence on the internet one of your first concerns should be the reliability of the website. Check the website address, the URL, for example. URLs that end in 'ac.uk' or 'edu' indicate that the page is part of a site that belongs to an academic institution such as a university: 'ac' stands for 'academic' and 'edu' is short for education. Similarly, 'gov' indicates a government site. In each case this gives you some confidence that the content will not be inaccurate or misleading. This is not sufficient in itself and you should carry out other checks.

- Can you identify the author of the content?
- Does the page include information about the date it was last updated or altered?
- Does the page give a list of references for its material, or links to other pages that can support it?

If the answer to any of these questions is no, and the site does not belong to a recognised organisation, then you should be careful about accepting the information it provides.

## SUMMARY

Health and social care research evidence is now more accessible than it has ever been. You can read papers on the internet 24 hours a day, you can search for research findings and be presented with thousands of papers in a matter of seconds and your patients and clients and their relatives can do the same. But this situation brings its own problems. There is too much research out there for one person to be familiar with all of it, many of the findings are contradictory and the quality of published research papers is not always as high as it should be.

Contemporary health and social care practitioners cannot simply adopt findings from one research report. They must take evidence from a range of research reports and from other sources as well. They need to blend this evidence with their own practice experience, with the expectations of their patients and clients and with an understanding of the environment in which they work. Evidence-based practice is not an easy option. In Part Two we will be discussing the skills and knowledge you need to be able to deliver evidence-based practice.

---

## KEY LEARNING POINTS

- Research projects in health and social care rarely establish 100% proof. However, over time a body of research can establish evidence with increasing accuracy.
- Three factors limit the accuracy of health and social care research: quality of design, quality of execution and the nature of the subject-matter.
- Disseminating, or communicating about, research findings is the final stage of the process: a project is not complete until its findings are made known.
- The publication process helps to ensure that published findings are honest and reliable, but it is not a perfect system.
- An understanding of the publication process helps the potential user of findings to understand the limitations of published papers.

---

## FURTHER READING

The first two references are internet journals: they are worth exploring as examples of the use of new technologies in the communication of research findings. The third reference is a difficult text, but it offers some very original insights into social science research.

*Early Childhood Research and Practice* **http://ecrp.uiuc.edu/**

*Internet Journal of Allied Health Sciences and Practice* **http://ijahsp.nova.edu/**

Starbuck, WH (2006) *The production of knowledge. The challenge of social science research*. Oxford: Oxford University Press

# Part Two

# Evidence-based Practice

Chapter 8

# Reviewing the Evidence

This chapter discusses the following topics.

- Applying evidence to practice.

- How can we judge relevance and applicability?

- Making use of research synthesis.

- Judging practical significance.

- Other sources of evidence.

## INTRODUCTION

I hope that Part One has helped you to understand the research process, the ways in which research evidence is created and the ways in which researchers let the rest of us know about their work. In this part we will concentrate on how practitioners can best make use of this work. A detailed discussion of practice development and change can be found in many other sources (see, for example, Jones, 2007; Hayes, 2007; Holbeche, 2006). Change theory, management theory and organisational theory are all concerned at least in part with how evidence is used to develop practice, but they are not subjects that I wish to dwell on here. What I do want to concentrate on are the more practical issues surrounding evidence-based practice, which are likely to have a direct impact on your work as a health or social care practitioner.

In this chapter we will look specifically at the importance of appraising the relevance and applicability of research evidence and at the role that **systematic reviews** can play in this process.

## RELIABLE, VALID, RELEVANT AND APPLICABLE?

In Part One I emphasised the importance of **reliability** and **validity** in research. You might remember that naturalistic researchers refer to these concepts as 'truthfulness' and 'transferability' but to make this discussion as clear as possible I will use 'reliability' and 'validity' to apply to all forms of health and social care research.

Reliability and validity are key qualities of research. Unreliable or invalid methods or designs result in poor-quality research whose findings have no credibility. But if you want to use research findings in developing evidence-based practice there are two other valuable criteria that you need to apply: relevance and applicability. Figure 1 illustrates the relationship between these criteria.

## RELEVANCE AND APPLICABILITY

A research project that is valid and reliable is not always relevant. An unreliable or invalid study is never relevant. A relevant study can be linked directly to your practice, informing that practice and also decisions about the way in which you may wish to develop it in the future. But that does not necessarily mean that the study can be used to initiate or support changes to practice. If you can use a study for these purposes then it is relevant *and* applicable.

For example, a study of children's experiences of hospitalisation might be reliable and valid. Despite this, a social worker for older people is unlikely to find it relevant or applicable. A social worker in children's services might find it relevant, but not directly applicable. A children's ward staff nurse, however, is likely to find it both relevant and applicable.

There is another distinction I want to make between these two pairs of characteristics. This relates to the issue of the age of research projects. Most writers will suggest to students that a literature review should always begin by searching for recent research papers, perhaps going back no more than four or five years. Many students seem to think that this is because

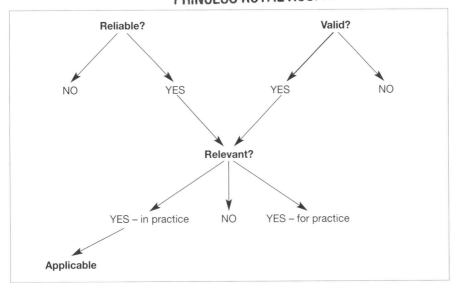

**Figure 1** Reliability, validity, relevance and applicability – links between the concepts

older research is no longer valid or reliable. This is not the case. Validity and reliability are not affected by the age of a paper: relevance and applicability are affected. If a research study was carried out correctly, using appropriate study design, methods and tools, then it remains valid and reliable. Things change, however, and the passing of time might well result in the focus of a study no longer being part of health or social care practice. As a result, a study that was once relevant to practice may become irrelevant, but this does not make it invalid or unreliable.

Even if you judge a study to be reliable, valid, relevant and applicable, will you act on its findings and change your practice? How much faith can be placed in a single piece of research?

## Key Question 1

An experimental, quantitative, study of 12 subjects who all have disease X finds that there is a slightly increased risk of problem A in this group compared to the general population.

- Would you be happy to make major changes to health care practice based on this study?
- What might make you feel confident about making these changes?
- What might make you concerned about basing changes on this single study?

My own experience leads me to believe that there are few occasions when I would recommend a change in practice based on the results of a single research project. A flawless research project is a rare thing indeed: there is usually something that could have been done more effectively, or a different choice of data analysis methods that would give slightly different results, or a **confidence interval** that is not quite what we would like.

Sometimes a single study does have an impact on practice well beyond what we might expect. I used an example as a basis for the study outline in Key Question 1: a paper published in 1998 by Wakefield *et al*. This paper reported on a study of children diagnosed with autistic spectrum disorder (ASD) and the results were reported in the media as 'proving' a link between ASD and the measles, mumps and rubella (MMR) vaccine. As a result of this study and its attendant publicity the MMR vaccination programme in the UK was severely affected. Many parents decided that the results of the study meant that their children were at risk of autism if they were given the MMR, or 'Triple', vaccination.

The original study was small. It investigated 12 children, 11 boys and one girl. Each child had developed developmental problems as well as gastroenterological problems such as abdominal pain. In eight of the children the parents associated the onset of behavioural symptoms with the administration of the MMR vaccine. In one case this onset was associated with the child developing measles. The study did not randomly select its subjects, nor did it use a **control group**. The debate about Wakefield *et al*'s results quickly began, with other studies and letters in the columns of medical journals appearing soon after. To some extent the debate continues and many parents remain concerned about the potential outcome of MMR vaccination.

Of course, in many cases if we read two or three research reports on the same subject we will get two or three different sets of results, leading to two or three different recommendations for change. In such circumstances what the busy health and social care practitioner needs is access to a research methodology that can offer more accurate evidence.

## RESEARCH SYNTHESIS

Making sense of a series of research reports can seem like a daunting task, even for experienced practitioners. But in some cases someone else will have done the work already, by undertaking research synthesis. This involves gathering together a group of research papers and re-analysing their findings to produce a single, much larger, research study. This study will hopefully provide a set of findings which is more accurate than those of each of the individual studies. If a statistical test can be applied to all of the data taken from the individual studies this process is called meta-analysis.

This way of synthesising the results of different studies is usually referred to as **systematic review**. Two organisations in health and social care are generally known for producing high-quality systematic reviews: in health care, the Cochrane Collaboration (**www.cochrane.org**) and in social care, the Campbell Collaboration (**www.campbellcollaboration.org**). These two organisations produce systematic reviews in similar ways and they will also work in partnership to develop review methods. Both of them also publish their reviews online.

Systematic reviews, as you might remember from Chapter 3, are at the top of the research hierarchy in health and social care. They are considered to offer the most reliable evidence for the effectiveness of interventions. But they are by no means perfect. Systematic reviews are only as good as the data available to them and if the body of original research is of poor quality then a systematic review will struggle to produce reliable results. You also need to be aware of what types of research evidence a systematic review uses. Many reviews, including those in the Cochrane Library, exclude naturalistic, qualitative, evidence. This means that reviews of socially-complex interventions, such as specialist nursing or social care interventions, may exclude the majority of sources of evidence on their subjects.

## Making sense of a systematic review

Systematic reviews differ from general literature reviews in a number of key ways:

- they have a much narrower focus;
- they aim to answer specific research questions;
- they undertake comprehensive searches for *all* the available research on the topic;
- they re-analyse the findings of each of the studies they review and in some cases obtain and re-analyse the original data collected from individual subjects.

Campbell and Cochrane reviews also share a specific approach to creating review questions and titles. Essentially, the review title *is* the question, but phrased as a brief statement. This approach means that a basic question such as 'How effective is single-dose oral aspirin for the treatment of lower back pain?' will become 'Single-dose oral aspirin for lower back pain' as the review title. A more complex question, perhaps comparing two interventions, might be: 'Which intervention, A or B, is more effective in treating problem C'. The review title then becomes 'A or B in the treatment of C'. Key Case 1 offers some examples.

## KEY CASE 1 – Systematic reviews

Cochrane Collaboration:

- Beta-blockers for hypertension;
- Family-centred care for children in hospital;
- School feeding for improving the physical and psychosocial health of disadvantaged elementary school children.

Campbell Collaboration:

- Case management for persons with substance use disorders;
- Effectiveness of offender management systems in the delivery of correctional services;
- Peer assisted learning for academic achievement in elementary school students.

## Literature searches in systematic reviews

Literature searches in systematic reviews take the ideas of sensitivity and specificity to their extremes. Once inclusion and exclusion criteria are identified a search will be undertaken of all appropriate databases using a detailed strategy and without setting time constraints on publication dates. Such a search will typically generate thousands of potentially relevant references which must each be considered during the second stage of the search. This second stage eliminates almost all the papers, as the inclusion and exclusion criteria are strictly applied.

## Assessing study quality

The shortlisted studies that have survived the initial selection process must be assessed for quality. Unlike general literature reviews, when study results are often reported with little consideration of the quality of the study design, systematic reviews will include only research which meets an objective quality assessment.

There are many tools that can be used to assess the qualities of studies being considered for inclusion in a systematic review, most of which have been developed to assess **experimental** study designs. One of the most widely used is the Jadad Score, or Scale (Bhogal *et al*, 2005). This is a straightforward tool for the assessment of trial reports which awards up to five points based on a study's use of **randomisation** and **blinding** and on its reporting of dropout and withdrawal. The Jadad Score has the advantage of being easy and quick to use, but it focuses on three very specific aspects of study design and reporting. It places great emphasis on **double-blinding**, for example, so that studies that cannot be double-blinded will score zero for this even if they use the level of blinding that is appropriate for the intervention being studied.

The EPOC checklist, developed by the Cochrane Collaboration Effective Practice and Organisation of Care review group (EPOC, 2002) is an example of a more complicated assessment tool. As with the Jadad Score, the EPOC checklist is designed to assess experimental studies but it does so by considering a far wider range of criteria. The checklist begins with a set of questions to judge whether a study meets the basic EPOC criteria for inclusion in a systematic review. If it doesn't then the assessment stops and the study is rejected. If the study is suitable for inclusion then a further nine sets of questions are applied, covering issues such as the interventions being studied, participant characteristics and project results.

A few 'discipline specific' tools have been developed. One example is the Physiotherapy Evidence-Based Database Scale (the PEDro Scale: Bhogal *et al*, 2005). The PEDro Scale uses ten quality criteria designed specifically to judge trials of physiotherapy interventions.

Each of these scales or scores is helpful in ensuring consistency of assessment across and between studies. However, the EPOC checklist and the PEDro Scale are not designed for novice researchers. They both demand knowledge of research design, experimental methodologies and statistical analysis.

All three of these examples focus on experimental studies. Assessment tools for naturalistic designs using qualitative methodologies are as yet much rarer, but groups such as the Cochrane Qualitative Research Methods Group are developing tools for this task.

Finally, after this stage of analysis is complete, a set of studies for inclusion will be established. This set is usually small, in low double figures at most. This is a reflection of the focused nature of systematic review questions or topics and of the strict inclusion criteria. It is also, at least in part, a reflection of the poor quality of many published research studies. In some cases a systematic review finds no studies that are suitable for inclusion: for example, a Cochrane Collaboration review on specialist epilepsy clinics which I co-authored (Bradley and Lindsay, 2001). These reviews are still of value to practitioners, as they help to establish the lack of evidence about a practice and so support the need for the carrying out of research in the future.

When a review does find studies worthy of inclusion then each study's methods and results need to be subjected to rigorous analysis. The extent of this analysis depends on factors such as the possibility of gaining access to the original data from each subject or participant, known as Individual Patient Data (IPD) in Cochrane reviews, or the degree of similarity in the outcomes measured by each study. If outcomes are similar and data is presented clearly then it may be possible to pool the individual studies' data and subject it to meta-analysis.

## Is there a systematic review to answer my question?

Unfortunately, I can't guarantee that there will be a systematic review to help with every health or social care question. Systematic reviews are relative newcomers, first developed in the late 1980s and early 1990s, and many important issues still have not been subject to high-quality systematic reviews. A large percentage of the first reviews produced by the Cochrane Collaboration focused on drug or surgical interventions and only in recent years has there been a move towards more reviews of complex interpersonal interventions, which are key parts of health and social care. So in many cases you will still need to undertake a research synthesis yourself.

---

**Key Question 2: Finding a systematic review**

Think of two or three practice issues you are currently interested in. Go online and search the Cochrane and Campbell libraries for systematic reviews on these subjects. If you find a relevant systematic review:

- What evidence does it use?
- What evidence does it exclude?

If you can't find a relevant systematic review:

- What reasons can you think of for this lack of a review?

---

## EVIDENCE FROM OTHER SOURCES

What do health and social care practitioners do when there is no research evidence, or at least no good-quality research evidence? Despite the vast amount of research that has been undertaken in the last 100 years it is surprisingly easy to meet a situation where research evidence can't give you the answers to your problems. So we have to find the evidence from other sources.

You may remember that definitions of evidence-based practice often refer to the use of 'best available evidence', not to the use of 'the best evidence there is, anywhere'. Health and social care practitioners regularly meet situations that have yet to attract researchers, or situations where the research evidence is far from clear. We also routinely find ourselves in acute situations that we are unfamiliar with but which require urgent action, giving us no time to check for research findings: a family in crisis or a cardiac arrest situation for example. And the nature of health and social care practice is such that we often have to deal with unique sets of circumstances which will never be explained by the application of research evidence. Because these situations and events are a routine part of health and social care practice we must always look for other sources of information that can act as the best available evidence for our actions.

## What else is 'evidence'?

Discussions about evidence-based practice (EBP) often refer to a time before it existed: a time when practice was based mainly on 'experience and judgement' (Clancy and Cronin, 2005, p.152). A reader could infer from this that experience and judgement are not evidence. But is this really the case? Should we dismiss experience and judgement, especially if they are based on decades of education and practice? I would hope that we don't. Health and social care has always been evidence based, the difference is that today we are no longer happy that the evidence used prior to the development of EBP can be classed as the best available. It is counter-productive to see 'research' and 'evidence' as synonymous. Yes, research is a source of evidence, but not all evidence comes from research. There are other sources of evidence: experience is just one of them.

Rycroft-Malone *et al* (2004, p.83) emphasise the need for EBP to use knowledge from more than one source, stressing that true EBP requires practitioners to 'draw on and integrate multiple sources of … knowledge informed by a variety of evidence bases that have been critically and publicly scrutinized'. They identify four such sources:

1  research;
2  clinical experience;
3  patients, clients and carers;
4  local context and environment (including audit and evaluation data, local professional networks, feedback from quality assurance programmes).

Gilgun (2005, p.52) presents a similar set of four sources for EBP in social care:

- research and theory;
- practice wisdom;
- 'the person of the practitioner' – personal assumptions and values;
- 'what clients bring to practice situations'.

## Key Question 3: Think of a recent problem in practice that you have solved.

Choosing either Rycroft-Malone *et al*'s or Gilgun's list of sources consider these questions.

- What combination of the four sources of evidence did you use to solve the problem?
- Which was the most valuable and why?
- Which was the least valuable and why?

To be able to draw on the knowledge provided by each source in order to create and deliver effective care requires skill and judgement: none of these sources is capable of meeting individuals' needs without the intervention of a skilled practitioner. Skilled practitioners know where to find evidence, how to make sense of it and how to appraise it. They also know how to apply it, and experience and judgement are central to this ability to apply evidence.

## KEY CASE 2 – Parachutes

If we rely solely on the use of evidence from **randomised controlled trials** and systematic reviews we will soon find that much health and social care practice is impossible to carry out. This is clearly shown by Smith and Pell (2003) in their paper on 'Parachute use to prevent death and major trauma related to gravitational challenge'.

As Smith and Pell note, parachutes are regularly used to prevent injury and death in falls from high altitude. However, their use does not prove effective in every case: they are not 100% reliable. Similarly, there are examples of individuals surviving falls from high altitude without a parachute: high-altitude falls are less than 100% fatal. Smith and Pell also note that the evidence for parachute use is generally low level, often no more than anecdote or single-case reports. There are no reports of randomised trials of parachute use.

If an intervention (the parachute) is known to be less than 100% effective and evidence for its use is of poor quality, should doctors not stop advocating its use until a high-quality trial is completed? If we keep strictly to the ideals of EBP then we could argue that doctors *should* stop recommending parachutes until their effectiveness is supported by objective evidence. If we apply common sense, the idea is clearly ridiculous. There are major practical issues, of recruitment at least, in setting up a randomised trial of parachute use. There are also ethical issues attached to such a risky research study. But above all, we don't need a randomised trial to tell us that parachutes are a good idea.

## ROLE OF THE SERVICE USER

Both Rycroft-Malone *et al* (2004) and Gilgun (2005) note the importance of the service user as a source of evidence. In Chapter 10 we will look at the service user's role in audit and evaluation, while in Chapter 11 we will discuss the developing importance of the service user in research. At this point I want to draw your attention to the active role that service user organisations can have in providing evidence for practice independent of these processes.

Service user organisations are becoming increasingly involved in the provision of evidence, as a development of their roles as user advisers, advocates or supporters. The most forward-thinking of these organisations realised some years ago that providing evidence for practitioners is one of the most effective ways of improving care for patients or clients. The advent of the internet has made this activity easier, as a well-designed website can reach health and social care practitioners across the world. Examples of this provision include Epilepsy Action (**www.epilepsy.org.uk**) and Diabetes UK (**www.diabetes.org.uk**), both of which have extensive resources for health and social care professionals. One of the best examples is the DIPEx project.

### KEY CASE 3: DIPEx

The DIPEx website can be found at **www.dipex.org**. DIPEx is a registered charity, established in 2001 by two doctors after they had both experienced health care as patients. Their professional backgrounds clearly informed their experiences, but it is as patients, or service users, that they approached the development of the charity. On the website, DIPEx provides 'interviews with everyday people about their own experiences of serious illness, health problems or health related matters' in the form of video and audio recordings. These interviews, which are categorised according to illness, condition or health-related issue, offer first-hand experiences of health care from service users of all ages and backgrounds. The information they give offers insights not only into the illnesses themselves but also into the social issues that the individuals have to deal with and into their relationships with health and social care professionals.

## SUMMARY

Health and social care involves decision-making: about the needs of individuals, communities or entire nations and the best ways of meeting these needs. Effective decision-making requires the best available evidence. Identifying this evidence is an often complicated process, but it's one which health and social care practitioners at all levels need to be able to undertake.

Once you have identified the best available evidence the next step is to use it. In Chapter 9 we will consider ways in which this can be done.

---

## KEY LEARNING POINTS

- Health and social care practice should be evidence based.
- Research provides much of this evidence, but it is not the only source.
- Experience, local knowledge and input from service users are also of value.
- Research evidence is the most important source of evidence for practice guidelines at organisational or national level.
- The care of individuals requires an evidence base incorporating all types of evidence.

---

## FURTHER READING

These three papers all discuss the nature of evidence in health and social care.

Gilgun, JF (2005) 'The four cornerstones of evidence-based practice in social work'. *Research on Social Work Practice*, 15: 52–61

Humphries, B (2003) 'What *else* counts as evidence in evidence-based social work?' *Social Work Education*, 22: 81–91

Rycroft-Malone, J, Seers, K, Titchen, A, Harvey, G, Kitson, A and McCormack, B (2004) 'What counts as evidence in evidence-based practice?' *Journal of Advanced Nursing*, 47: 81–90

**Chapter 9**

# Putting the Evidence into Practice

This chapter discusses the following topics.

- Using evidence to influence and change practice.

- Implementing findings and avoiding barriers.

- Using evidence for change on a large scale (global, national, organisational).

- Using evidence for personal or local change.

## INTRODUCTION

So far we have discussed the nature of evidence in health and social care, how that evidence is created, how it's communicated to health and social care practitioners and how we can judge its potential value. The end result of these processes should be the creation and identification of a body of evidence that is potentially of value to health and social care practice. In this chapter we will discuss the next stage: putting the evidence to use in influencing or changing practice.

## THE RELATIONSHIP BETWEEN EVIDENCE AND PRACTICE

If every health or social care professional agreed on what evidence is of value and also agreed on the ways in which this evidence should be used, this would be the simplest process so far. Unfortunately, health and social care practitioners rarely agree on the quality of evidence or on the best way to use it. Some of the most fundamental changes to health and social care practice have come about only after many years of argument and disagreement, while some changes that everyone agrees need to be made take years to be achieved because no-one can agree on the nature of these changes. Other changes to practice have been made in a short period of time, only for practitioners to decide later that they were unnecessary or undertaken in the wrong way.

> ### Key Question 1: Evidence-based change
>
> What evidence has created change in our approaches to these major health issues?
>
> - Smoking.
> - Sudden Infant Death and advice about babies' sleeping position.
> - Placing children in care.
> - Using mobile phones while driving.

A key point to remember is that evidence-based practice does not entail the use of evidence only to *change* practice. It can also involve the use of evidence to support existing practice: in other words, to argue *against* change. We will consider this use of evidence in Chapter 10, but please remember it as a legitimate and valuable use of evidence. Change is not the sole outcome of developing an evidence base. However, it is the outcome that we will be discussing in this chapter.

## TOP DOWN OR BOTTOM UP?

Evidence-based changes to practice can appear from two directions: bottom up or top down. In the top-down approach change is initiated at a high level, filtering through the lower levels until it impacts directly on individual practitioners. In a bottom-up approach change begins at the level of the individual, team or small unit and gradually moves upwards through levels of management until, potentially, it is taken up at organisational, national or even international level.

Top-down change comes from a high level of management and is intended to create alterations to practice at lower levels. For example, a hospital Chief Executive might initiate changes to the shift patterns of ward nursing staff, or a Director of Social Services might want to implement a new system of record-keeping for care-home staff. At national level, a government department might introduce a new policy which is intended to affect health or social care practitioners across the country.

Those people who initiate change from the top might be seen to have a number of advantages that they can use to make sure that change does take place. They can call on a vast range of evidence. They have the resources to pay for research projects to produce evidence. They may have managerial responsibility and therefore a degree of power over those they want to influence. They are likely to have access to the media and to have the resources to produce material that they can use to promote their aims. But this is no guarantee of success.

If you want to initiate evidence-based change from the bottom up it might appear that you have a tougher struggle ahead. 'Grass roots' practitioners lack managerial power, resources, access to media or marketing strategies. They don't have communications officers or press and public relations departments that they can call on for support. But this does not mean that they are doomed to failure.

Change is far from straightforward and you can find examples of success-ful change from the bottom up as well as from the top down. You can also find examples of evidence-based change that arise from outside the man-agement hierarchies of health and social care: what might be called externally-driven change. In externally-driven change pressure arises from groups or individuals with strong motivation to create change, who can call on evidence to support their intentions and use it to gather support within the health and social care communities.

Voluntary organisations and charities can sometimes initiate change in this way. There are even examples of change where the initial drive has arisen from a single individual or family.

## Key Question 2: Consumer-led change

Choose a health or social care specialism. Visit the websites of the largest or best-known voluntary organisations within this specialism.

- What changes are these organisations currently supporting?
- How are they attempting to initiate these changes?
- How successful do you think they are in achieving their aims?

## How to implement evidence-based change

Change theories fill many large and complex textbooks. Detailed discus-sion is outside the scope of this book, but it is worth considering some of the strategies that can be used to create change in health and social care practice. Needham (2000) identifies six of these strategies.

1 *Passive dissemination*: publishing research findings, sending policy documents and guidelines to practitioners and managers.

2 *Education*: running conferences or workshops about new developments.
3 *Marketing*: actively promoting change to targeted groups or individuals who have the power to initiate these changes.
4 *Mass media*: creating a widespread awareness of the potential benefits of change and so creating informal pressure for its implementation.
5 *Performance management*: assessing the performance of a group or an individual and giving feedback to produce a change in their practice.
6 *Incentives*: rewards, such as promotion or pay awards, based on the achievement of targets.

## Key Question 3: Using change strategies

For each of Needham's six strategies, think of examples from health and social care.

- Which strategy has been most effective in your experience?
- Which strategy is the least effective?
- Do some of these strategies work particularly well in 'bottom-up' change?

## Barriers to change

Even if people agree that a change is a good idea it isn't always easy to introduce that change. When there is disagreement about the benefits of changing practice introducing change can be extremely difficult.

Change is often threatening. Health and social care practice has been subject to almost constant change in recent decades and as a result many practitioners are reluctant to alter their practice unless there is no alternative. Evidence that supports the way things are, the status quo, may be more readily accepted by practitioners than evidence that supports new practice.

## CHANGING PERSONAL PRACTICE

Creating a genuine, long-lasting, change in the practice of a group of people is daunting and difficult for even the most experienced practitioner. If you are inexperienced, lack managerial or political influence or resources it can be virtually impossible. However, any individual health or social care practitioner has the potential to change their personal practice to some degree. This can't, of course, simply be change for change's sake: neither can it be done suddenly. Changes to personal practice need to be evidence based. An ability to identify and appraise research and other evidence in order to identify findings that are relevant and applicable to your practice is critical. But what do you do if there is no identifiable evidence in support of your intended change? You can abandon your attempt, but for a well-motivated practitioner this is a frustrating outcome of the desire to improve care. Alternatively, you can seek to develop your own evidence, through practitioner inquiry.

## PRACTITIONER INQUIRY

Health and social care literature often discusses the concept of 'practitioner inquiry'. Shaw (2005, p.1232) describes this as 'evaluation, research, development, or more general inquiry that is small-scale, local, grounded, and carried out by professionals who directly deliver those self-same services'. In other words, it's a form of inquiry undertaken by practitioners about their own practice and that of their colleagues. The aim of this inquiry is to explore, explain and perhaps alter this practice to ensure that it is as effective as possible.

I am wary, as is Shaw, of differentiating inquiry by practitioners from investigations by anyone else, be they academics, managers or service users. If practitioner inquiry had its own unique aims, methods or code of ethics then I might have a different opinion, but it doesn't. Nonetheless, it is often written about as if it was somehow separate.

Investigation by practitioners into their own practice is sometimes referred to as 'insider research' to differentiate it from the more usual 'outsider research'. This is a more useful distinction to make than 'practitioner researcher' versus 'academic researcher'. Insider researchers, who are part of the situation, event or intervention under study, may have a different impact on the study than outsiders would have and would also be open to different potential **biases**. Insider researchers, for example, may be producing evidence on which their own jobs may depend.

Practitioner research or inquiry can be undertaken using any of the research methodologies we discussed in Chapter 3. Strongly **positivist**, **experimental**, **methodologies** such as randomised trials can be undertaken by practitioners, as can **interpretive**, **naturalistic**, studies. My reading of the practitioner research literature, however, suggests a strong emphasis on naturalistic, qualitative, approaches with an equally strong emphasis on self-reflection. This may be a reflection of the complexity and expense of reliable and valid positivist research designs, or of the focus of health and social care research on subjective experience as evidence. Whatever the reason, the result is that practitioner research texts in health and social care seem to neglect **quantitative data** and so close off a valuable source of evidence. In medicine, by contrast, there is a long history of practitioners developing and undertaking large-scale **randomised controlled trials** in co-operation with academic colleagues. Naturalistic practitioner research in medicine is still a minority activity, although it is slowly increasing.

It also seems to me that a high proportion of practitioner research is carried out as part of a course of study. Pre-registration or undergraduate students are usually required to carry out a small study, often a literature review or a case study. Masters students will carry out larger studies, which may be fieldwork based. Doctoral students, whose theses are expected to be up to 100,000 words in length, will carry out substantial original research projects in order to gain their qualifications.

Once completed, examined and awarded a 'pass' mark a high proportion of undergraduate and masters level practitioner research goes no further. Hopefully each of these studies will have increased its creator's knowledge, skills and understanding but it is unlikely that its direct influence on practice will extend much beyond this. Although many published research papers in health and social care stem from work undertaken to achieve a qualification, they still represent only a small proportion of this work.

One research methodology, action research, offers practitioners the opportunity to undertake research collaboratively, extending the likely influence of a study across a team of practitioner researchers.

## ACTION RESEARCH

Action research, according to Fox *et al* (2007, p.79), is 'a composite term for several research designs focusing on action leading to change'. Coghlan and Brannick (2005, p.3) suggest that four characteristics define the methodology:

1  research *in* action, rather than research *about* action;
2  a collaborative democratic partnership;
3  concurrent with action;
4  a sequence of events and an approach to problem-solving.

In other words, action researchers are part of the activity or situation being investigated. They work as a team, they study the activity or situation as it happens, and through a cyclical approach to research they can constantly initiate change, gather evidence, refine practice, gather further evidence, and so on, until genuine, effective and beneficial improvements to practice can be demonstrated. In this way action research resembles other processes in health and social care such as the nursing process or the audit cycle.

This focus on change is a key characteristic of action research. It is probably true to say that it's a defining characteristic of this methodology. If change isn't initiated and analysed then it isn't action research. Simply seeking to describe, explore or explain a phenomenon isn't good enough for the action researcher: the project must also alter the phenomenon and analyse the impact of this action.

The centrality of change also links into another characteristic of action research: it is focused on a specific setting or locality. This is referred to as 'immersion' in the research setting, as 'knowledge in action' and as the use of data which is 'contextually embedded and interpreted' (Coghlan and Brannick, 2005, p.7).

For many health and social care practitioners and academics the way in which action research focuses on change within a specific setting makes it a powerful research methodology. Action research offers a structured way of making changes, testing them and providing evidence for long-term decisions about their effectiveness. Change is not imposed from outside, or supported solely by research carried out somewhere else. Action research provides evidence gathered directly from the change within the service or locality that wants to adopt the change.

Action research's emphasis on collaboration and teamwork has been taken even further by researchers and practitioners who see most other methodologies as representing an imbalance of power. This imbalance is perceived as one that ensures that control of knowledge remains with 'expert' researchers, senior managers and funding organisations. To further correct this imbalance action research has been refined and two additional variations have been created: participatory action research and emancipatory research.

Once again, the introduction of new research methodologies does not necessarily make it easier to understand the ways in which investigations are carried out. However, the three variations can, I think, be broadly described as follows.

- *Action research*: a research process that seeks to investigate, understand and change a situation or activity on a local level. An 'expert' researcher may lead this process, with the involvement of the practitioners being studied.
- *Participatory action research (PAR)*: removes the idea of the 'expert researcher' and removes the distinction between researcher and practitioner. Practitioners lead the process, taking advice when necessary but ensuring that they retain control of the action research cycle (Fox *et al*, 2007).

- *Emancipatory research (ER)*: focuses on marginalised or disempowered social groups. It is a process that aims to change others' perceptions of these groups and also aims to change the perceptions of group members in a positive, empowering, way (Fox *et al*, 2007).

There are other interpretations of course. Coupland and Maher (2005, p.191) state that PAR, rather than ER, is a '"bottom up" approach that seeks to empower affected communities'. In their PAR project with young injecting drug users the research was undertaken as a collaboration between academic researchers, health workers and 'peer workers' who were either ex-drug users or in close contact with users. Interestingly, neither the peer workers nor the drug users had any input into the design of the study. Coupland and Maher state that the health workers would not carry out data collection outside their normal working hours so the academics and peer workers did most of the data collection at these times. In addition, the peer workers were selected by the researchers and the health workers were selected by their managers: the young drug users seem to have had no say in this selection. Peer worker involvement is referred to by the researchers as 'work experience', which suggests that they were not paid for their activities: there is no mention in the paper of what payments were made to the peer workers. You might question who exactly was 'empowered' by these strategies.

Action research appears to be the answer to a health or social care practitioner's needs. It puts practitioners in control of the research process. It eliminates the presence of the outsider researcher, with all the problems such a person might create in an organisation. Everyone in the situation gets a say about how the research is carried out. It's an ongoing process which creates evidence, acts on that evidence and then refines it on the basis of the study of the changed or altered practice. It seems to be an ideal way for a team or small organisation to create and use its own evidence for practice.

Unfortunately, action research is no more straightforward than any of the more established methodologies. It has developed over the last 60 years from the early work of Kurt Lewin and others and has been influenced by a variety of schools of thought, including Marxism and feminism (Coghlan and Brannick, 2005). It has developed its own often impenetrable jargon and has been expanded, re-organised and subdivided by numerous authors. As a result it is difficult to understand exactly what researchers mean when they use the term 'action research'. It is a term that causes a lot of confusion in the minds of health and social care practitioners and researchers (Fox *et al*, 2007). In addition to, and partly because of, this confusion action research's standing within the broader research community is limited. Action research has 'at best, ambiguous standing in the research world' and in the academic world its standing is 'limited' (Fox *et al*, 2007, p.48).

Part of the problem with action research is the separation between its practice and the rhetoric of the action research literature. Many research projects are labelled as action research even though they fail to display the required characteristics. In some cases the label is used simply because the research is being undertaken by a practitioner, in other cases it is used even though there is no evidence of a cyclical approach and in others it seems to be used to describe any project that undertakes fieldwork or observation in a practice area.

Because of these variations in definition and approach you need to be very clear about what researchers mean when they describe their work as 'action research'. Action research does offer practitioners a set of strategies for studying and improving their own practice but it is not the straightforward, empowering, research methodology that some authors would claim.

## SUMMARY

Using evidence to influence, develop or change practice is a complex activity. Change management needs more than just a body of supporting evidence, for there are barriers to change that can seem insurmountable even when the evidence for change is unchallenged. For the junior or inexperienced practitioner the introduction of large-scale change may be too big a task, but evidence-based changes to personal practice can be achieved.

Practitioner inquiry, particularly through action research, offers practitioners a series of ways of creating a body of evidence for change. In these approaches to research, data is gathered within the local context and offers direct evidence about local practice. This type of evidence is often seen by practitioners as more 'real' than evidence gathered elsewhere. Using this type of evidence can offer a higher likelihood of success in initiating change.

---

### KEY LEARNING POINTS

- Good-quality evidence is always needed to support changes in practice.
- Changes to personal practice need evidence to support them however small or minor these changes may appear.
- Practitioner inquiry enables evidence for practice to be gathered locally, by insiders, rather than imposed on practitioners from outside.
- Action research is a key methodology for practitioner inquiry but the term can be misused.

---

## FURTHER READING

Clancy, CM and Cronin, K (2005) 'Evidence-based decision making: global evidence, local decisions'. *Health Affairs*, 24: 151–62

Fox, M, Martin, P and Green, G (2007) *Doing practitioner research*. London: Sage

Shaw, I (2005) 'Practitioner research: evidence or critique?' *British Journal of Social Work*, 35: 1231–48

Smith, GCS and Pell, JP (2003) 'Parachute use to prevent death and major trauma related to gravitational challenge: systematic review of randomised controlled trials'. *British Medical Journal*, 327: 1459–61. Don't take this paper seriously. It shows just how ridiculous care delivery can become if we stick rigidly to the idea that randomised trials are always the best form of evidence.

## Chapter 10

# Audit and Evaluation

This chapter discusses the following topics.

- Ensuring effective practice through audit and evaluation.

- Defining and differentiating audit, evaluation and research.

- When do you audit?

- When do you evaluate?

- Service user involvement in audit and evaluation.

## INTRODUCTION

Audit and evaluation are common activities in health and social care. But despite their now established places many practitioners, managers and academics seem to have trouble telling the two apart and differentiating them from research.

In this chapter we will consider the roles of audit and evaluation in health and social care, define each of the activities and decide on the differences between audit and evaluation and research. These differences are not just theoretical ones, they also have practical and ethical implications for practitioners, clients and patients.

## AUDIT AND EVALUATION: WHAT ARE THEY?

> ### Key Question 1 – Audit and evaluation
>
> What do these words mean to you in terms of:
>
> - the activities they describe;
> - when these activities take place;
> - what impact they can have on practice?

Audit and evaluation are part of quality assurance. They are two related strategies for the measurement of service provision that help practitioners to understand what standard of care they are achieving (Gomm and Davies, 2000). In other words, they are both ways of providing evidence about current practice. Although research can do this, audit and evaluation provide evidence in ways that have certain characteristics that are different from research.

## DIFFERENTIATING AUDIT, EVALUATION AND RESEARCH

The clearest way to differentiate audit and evaluation, in my experience, is that suggested by the COREC Ethics Consultation E-Group (2006). This group, set up by the Central Office of Research Ethics Committees (COREC, renamed the National Research Ethics Service in April 2007) with the aim of informing decisions about ethics committee approval, concluded that neither audit nor evaluation projects needed to gain the approval of a research ethics committee. A critical reason for this is that both audit and evaluation measure *current practice*. They do not introduce or test new practices and they do not require patients or clients to receive untried interventions. Research, by contrast, has more complex and wide ranging aims. It seeks to produce generalisable or transferable new knowledge, to generate hypotheses or to develop and test theories.

The E-Group also established other criteria for telling the difference between audit and evaluation.

Audit:

- is designed to answer the question 'Does this service reach a predetermined standard?';
- measures against this pre-determined standard;
- measures an intervention in current use;

- analyses existing data, or collects basic additional data (for example, through a questionnaire);
- does not involve the use of **intervention** or **control groups**: there is no **randomisation**.

Evaluation:

- is designed to answer the question 'What standard does this service achieve?';
- measures current service without reference to a pre-determined standard;
- measures an intervention in current use;
- analyses existing data, or collects basic additional data (for example, through a questionnaire);
- does not involve the use of intervention or control groups: there is no randomisation.

Research, on the other hand:

- is exploratory or experimental;
- seeks explanations for its findings;
- introduces new and untried interventions and hence risk;
- may need to collect additional data, or subject patients or clients to additional interventions, beyond those which are necessary for the person's care.

With these criteria in mind you should find it relatively easy to differentiate audit or evaluation from research. Using the first two criteria, you should be able to differentiate audit from evaluation.

Audit and evaluation have also been referred to as ways of providing 'knowledge from local context' (Rycroft-Malone *et al*, 2004, p.86). This is a useful additional way of distinguishing them from research. Research evidence can be created at a local level, but it can also be brought in from other locations, potentially from the other side of the world. Research has the potential to be generalisable or transferable: audit and evaluation data are of most use to the services within which the data was collected.

What audit and evaluation don't do:

- they don't necessarily measure against best available evidence;
- they don't demonstrate that the standard achieved is the best possible standard;
- they don't automatically enable comparison with services from other providers;
- they tell us what standard is to be achieved but not how to achieve it.

## Other definitions

The COREC criteria are useful, but there are other definitions and descriptions that you might find helpful. Alcolado and Bennett (2006, p.491) distinguish audit from research because audit 'involves no experimental intervention and it compares observed practice to recognised guidelines or protocols'. Morrison (2003, p.385) emphasises that evaluation is focused on 'local quality improvement'. Jamtvedt *et al* (2006) define an audit as a summary of the performance of care during a given time period. These definitions, as well as others, agree on many key aspects of audit and evaluation. They tend to view both activities as focusing on local care provision, as measuring existing accepted practices and as not exposing patients, clients or carers to untested interventions. But there is still enough disagreement among health and social care practitioners to leave even experienced individuals confused about the differences between audit, evaluation and research.

Morrison (2003, p.385), writing specifically about medicine, states that evaluation 'is analogous to clinical audit'. Prideaux and Rogers (2006, p.498) note that 'the dividing line between research and audit is subject to considerable variation'. They suggest that some NHS Ethics Committees have so little understanding of non-biomedical, non-experimental, research that they automatically classify all of it as 'audit', removing the need for ethical approval. I would have agreed with this a few years ago, but I think NHS Ethics Committees have extended their knowledge in recent years.

Social care professionals can also add to the confusion. In his review of a mixed methods study of counselling in schools, Hanley (2006, p.150) declares that the report 'covered all the bases for a good piece of research, and was exactly what it said it was in the title (an evaluation report)'. Other authors refer to their projects as 'evaluative research' (Waldman, 2005; McCarthy, 2000).

With such confusion over the exact nature of audit, evaluation and research being expressed by experienced professionals and academics it's not surprising that students and inexperienced practitioners should have problems telling them apart. When you read a report it's worth giving some thought to the nature of the activity being discussed, whether or not the report declares it to be audit, evaluation or research. But the most important consideration is of the project's quality. If the work is not valid or reliable then it is of little value to your practice, whatever type of work it is.

## WHEN TO AUDIT OR EVALUATE

From the definitions of audit and evaluation that I chose earlier, it's clear that both audit and evaluation take place in specific circumstances.

- Audit needs pre-determined standards to be in place: you need to measure practice against these standards.
- Evaluation enables you to measure performance so that standards can be set.

So if you have a new or changed aspect of practice and you want to assess the standard it is achieving, then you will need to undertake an evaluation. If you already have standards for a practice activity, then an audit will enable you to judge if these standards are being met. Areas of practice that should have standards identified are known as performance indicators (PI). PIs tell you what should be measured: the standard lets you know what level of achievement is required for each PI.

Standards are not always applied locally, of course. Care standards are increasingly being applied much more broadly, through their establishment by voluntary organisations, professional organisations or government departments at a regional, national or international level (see, for example, Smith *et al*, 2007).

## WHAT STANDARDS MATTER?

Hopefully, every standard matters. However, there is always the possibility that standards used to measure performance don't measure *relevant* performance. For example, the fact that every patient is seen within ten minutes of arrival at a clinic is a readily measurable indicator of the speed at which the clinic functions, but it tells me little about how effectively the clinic functions.

Every patient might well be seen within ten minutes, but this may be achieved in Clinic 1 by limiting consultations to five minutes each. As a result, a typical patient may need three appointments before a satisfactory outcome is achieved. Clinic 2 may see only 50% of patients within ten minutes of arrival, but may typically achieve a satisfactory result on the first visit. If the only standard measured is the 'waiting time' standard, Clinic 2 performs poorly compared to Clinic 1. If 'time to satisfactory outcome' was measured, Clinic 2 would come out on top. If you were the patient, which of these standards would matter to you?

## KEY CASE 1 – Developing standards

In their development of PIs for the primary care of children with epilepsy, Caplin *et al* (2006) showed how standards can be established through a process of research review and expert evaluation on a national level. The team set out to establish PIs based on best available evidence evaluated by a panel of experts in the field, using a method known as the Delphi Technique. Their first activity involved the development of a set of 68 draft PIs based on a detailed review of research evidence. Each draft PI was supported by specific research findings. Once the draft PIs were established a panel of 13 experts in the treatment and care of children with epilepsy were asked to rate the importance of each PI. Those PIs which at least 80% of the panel rated as of highest importance were incorporated in the final set of standards. This final set consisted of 30 PIs, each of which was defined in clear, measurable, terms.

There are areas of Caplin *et al*'s study that can be criticised. The way in which 'expertise' was defined in order to select the panel was heavily biased towards doctors and behavioural scientists: there were no nurses or social workers, for example. Although the group that drafted the first set of PIs did include three parents, there were no parents in the 'expert' group that had the final say and at no time were children consulted. However, the process does clearly illustrate how standards or PIs can be developed at a national level, using the best available research evidence coupled with clinical expertise, to create a set of understandable and achievable measures that can be applied to a range of services, enabling the resulting audits to provide comparative information.

## Key Question 2: Standards and achievement

An audit report on a local service is sent to you for comment. Some of the standards and the scores achieved by the service are as follows.

- Clients will be seen within 30 minutes of arrival at reception. Target – 90%. Achieved – 75%.
- Clients will see the same practitioner at each visit. Target – 95%. Achieved – 95%.
- Clients will be given four consultations at most. Target – 100%. Achieved – 100%.
- Practitioners will work no more than 48 hours per week. Target – 100%. Achieved – 65%.

Are these standards all of equal importance?

Which result concerns you the most, if any?

What do these standards tell you about the outcomes of this service?

## INVOLVING SERVICE USERS IN AUDIT AND EVALUATION

There is a strong and growing body of opinion that regards the role of service users in audit or evaluation as being of vital importance (Humphries, 2003: Rycroft-Malone *et al*, 2004). This is part of a much wider movement towards the involvement of service users in the overall planning and development of health and social care services. The idea that service users should be involved in these activities has been accepted for some years (Telford and Faulkner, 2004). In 1999 the Department of Health published *Patient and Public Involvement in the New NHS*, which emphasised the importance of this involvement, and there seems to be little opposition to it within the literature. I will discuss service user involvement in research in the next chapter. In this chapter I want to dis-cuss service user involvement in audit and evaluation.

Although the idea of service user involvement in planning and developing services is now well-established, the practice is not as widespread as many people had hoped. There is little evidence that user involvement is becoming commonplace in the NHS (Telford and Faulkner, 2004) while in social care the involvement of service users remains firmly in the control of the service's managers and professionals (Beresford and Croft, 2001). This doesn't mean that service user involvement initiatives have failed: indeed, you could argue that any level of service user involvement is an improvement on the situation before the late 1990s. But it does mean that service user involvement is rarely as influential or empowering as its proponents would have us believe. As with many of the concepts we have already discussed, you should always read critically any report that claims service user involvement.

Individual patients, clients or carers are most likely to be involved in health and social care planning and development through participation in audit or evaluation. In both of these processes patients, clients or carers might be asked to take part by completing questionnaires, being inter-viewed or joining focus groups. This participation is potentially extremely valuable. In the development of standards the opinion of service users can provide evidence for which standards are important and for what level of performance might be expected within a standard. Once standards are established, service user participation in the audit process can provide key information about the service's ability to meet the standards.

At a more strategic level, service user organisations can be directly involved in developing entire processes for audit or evaluation. In some cases these processes are simply guidelines for service users to give them some idea of what constitutes an acceptable level of care provision. In other cases service user organisations can produce high-quality systems that can be adopted by, or at least can substantially inform, the audit and evaluation activities of provider organisations.

Service user involvement is not completely problem free and you should always be cautious of audit or evaluation processes that focus too much on the perceptions of service users. Two problems in particular can arise: over-involvement and inexperience.

Over-involvement of individual patients, clients or carers can arise when the service being audited or evaluated deals with a small number of users, or where service users have a long-term relationship with the service. It can also arise if a service is newly-established or is innovative and hence is subject to greater than usual scrutiny. In each of these cases service users may be asked for their input into quality assurance more frequently than usual. Some people will refuse if they feel that they do not wish to participate but others may feel obliged to take part even if they don't want to. This is a problem that can be avoided by careful consideration of who is asked to participate and by developing clear guidance about service user involvement.

Service user inexperience can lead to a contrasting problem. Rather than relying on the over-use of a small number of people with a high degree of involvement with a service, audit or evaluation may be based on the perception of people who have little involvement with or understanding of a service. This leads to the gathering of data about relatively superficial aspects of a service, or results in respondents making judgements based on limited understanding. Evaluating a service in this way is unreliable and presenting the results of such an approach can mislead.

## Key Question 3: Judging service quality

Imagine that you own an electrical item which breaks down. You take it to a repairer to be mended. The repairer takes a quick look, tells you that it will take two weeks to repair and will cost up to £100. It's an important item and will cost over £500 to replace, so you agree. After all, you don't really understand how it works or what needs fixing.

Ten days later the repairer calls. The item is fixed, a new part has been fitted and the bill is only £80. A good result, but ask yourself these questions.

- Did it really take ten days to fix, or did it lie on the shelf for nine days until the repairer started work on it?
- Was it really going to cost £100 to repair?
- Did it actually cost as much as £80?
- How can you tell if it has a brand-new part fitted, or if the old part has been mended?

Many people who access health or social care services are in a similar position. They understand little about how these services work, what they do or what alternative services they might have chosen. They may well have valid and insightful views of these services, but with regard to many critical areas of care they have little knowledge or understanding. Their ability to judge service quality is affected to a large extent by their understanding and so while they can offer valid insights into things that they are familiar with in everyday life, such as the quality of food or the friendliness of staff, many aspects of health and social care have no everyday equivalents on which to base comparisons.

In my experience, health and social care professionals generally view the principles of audit and evaluation positively. We want to do the best possible job and having clear and unambiguous standards to reach gives us an objective measure of success. However, both health and social services are often seen as overly bureaucratic, with a heavy reliance on audit or evaluation processes that are poorly designed and lack the desired clarity.

An additional complaint about audit and evaluation is that they do not always feed back results to the practitioners who have been assessed. If you don't know how you are performing, it is argued, then you can't improve your practice effectively. Interestingly, a Cochrane **systematic review** (Jamtvedt *et al*, 2006) found that while audit and feedback can improve professional practice the effect is generally small or moderate. Feedback effectiveness was highest when practice quality was low, probably because in this type of situation there is more room for improvement than in situations where practice standards are high.

## SUMMARY

Audit and evaluation are crucial activities for the provision of evidence about current practice. Although they may appear to be the responsibility of managers, practitioners must understand how these activities work and must be able to critically appraise the results of audit and evaluation to see how they apply to practice. Audit and evaluation data can help us to develop and improve practice but only if the standards set and measured are reliable and relevant.

KEY LEARNING POINTS

- Audit, evaluation and research are separate activities but the differences between them are not always clear.
- The effectiveness of audit and evaluation depends on factors such as appropriate standards, reliable data collection and analysis, and clear feedback.
- Service users have an important role to play in audit and evaluation but you need to make sure that their involvement isn't merely 'window dressing'.

## FURTHER READING

COREC Ethics Consultation E-Group (2006) *Differentiating audit, service evaluation and research*. **www.nres.npsa.nhs.uk/applicants/help/guidance. htm#audit** (20 June 2007)

Jamtvedt, G, Young, JM, Kristoffersen, DT, O'Brien, MA and Oxman, AD (2006) 'Audit and feedback: effects on professional practice and health care outcomes'. *Cochrane Database of Systematic Reviews*, issue 2

Morrison, J (2003) 'ABC of learning and teaching in medicine: evaluation'. *British Medical Journal*, 326: 385–7

Prideaux, D and Rogers, W (2006) 'Audit or research: the ethics of publication'. *Medical Education*, 40: 497–9

# Chapter 11

# 'Closing the Circle': Issues for the Future

This chapter discusses the question: 'what are the issues of importance in the development of research and evidence-based practice?'

• Speed of change in health and social care.

• New and forthcoming developments.

• International nature of health and social care.

• Will I have to do research?

• Service user involvement.

## INTRODUCTION

This textbook, like textbooks in general, has spent most of its time looking back. I have made use of the ideas of many other authors, discussed research projects that have already happened and referred to policies and procedures from years gone by. This tendency to look to the past is also a central feature of research, audit and evaluation. When you read a research report you are reading about data that was collected months, or even years, before the paper was published. Audit measures care against standards that already exist. Evaluation makes judgements about care that has already taken place.

You might wish to argue, of course, that research is as much about predicting future events as it is about judging past ones. This is true to some extent, but in health and social care researchers' predictions are usually conservative and based on cautious analysis of the data. The wilder predictions about the future of health and social care are often the result of media speculation. For the rest of this chapter, I will attempt some predictions of my own.

## THE SPEED OF CHANGE

In recent decades both health and social care have been characterised by change, in the UK and internationally. Individual changes are too numerous to list, but even a few minutes of thought should allow you to think of examples.

### Key Question 1 – Changes in health and social care

What examples can you think of? On your own, or with friends or colleagues, think about changes in the last ten years in areas such as:

- new drugs;
- new policies;
- new practices;
- role development;
- any other aspect of health and social care that you can think of.

Health and social care do not exist in isolation. Much of the research we have considered in this book has been research into health and social care undertaken by health and social care professionals and academics. It is certainly true that this research has a big impact on the practice of health and social care, but it is not the only influence. Health and social care is located within the societies and communities it serves and it is influenced as much by changes in these environments as it is by internal factors.

I expect that most of you reading this book will be relatively young and your direct experiences of health and social care will go back no more than 20 or 30 years, mostly as patients in primary care. From this rather brief experience you might find it hard to remember that contemporary health and social care provision is fairly young itself. While we can trace many aspects of health and social care back to the mid-nineteenth century, or even earlier, the provision of health and social care through national systems, funded through taxation and managed through central or local government, is decades, not centuries, old. The National Health Service (NHS) was created in 1948, for example, and even within its 60 year lifetime it has undergone many reorganisations.

Before state-controlled health and social care became the norm much of this care was provided by religious groups, voluntary organisations and charities. It was funded by donations or by insurance schemes, or by direct payments from patients or clients to the practitioners. In the twenty-first century we can see many examples of state-controlled health and social care moving once again into the remit of charities or the private sector. Society's view of health and social care is changing yet again.

In the last quarter of the twentieth century we also witnessed massive technological changes that led to new ways of managing and delivering care. Two of these changes in particular are worth considering: the creation and expansion of personal computing and the development of mobile communication technology. Taken together these two changes have had a major impact on health and social care in less than 20 years. They have revolutionised health and social care delivery, the way in which practitioners work and the ways in which they are educated and trained. They have also revolutionised the way in which many patients and clients interact with health and social care services and practitioners.

# NEW AND FORTHCOMING DEVELOPMENTS

Hopefully, when you think about factors that have created change in the past you can see how these factors interacted with health and social care to result in the care services we have today. But it is also crucial that you understand that these change processes will continue. We have not yet, and possibly never will have, reached a position where any aspect of health and social care is finalised.

## Health and social care: a SWOT analysis

SWOT stands for Strengths, Weaknesses, Opportunities and Threats. So a SWOT analysis is a way of analysing something, whether it's an individual, a business organisation or a large-scale service, to identify what its strengths, weaknesses, opportunities and threats might be. Figure 1 shows my informal, subjective, SWOT analysis of health and social care, written in early 2007.

| Strengths | Weaknesses |
|---|---|
| • Popular with the community<br>• Generally viewed as successful<br>• Has a committed, skilled, workforce<br>• Provides effective therapeutic care | • Limited resources<br>• Specific failures or perceived failures can have a large negative impact<br>• Extremely bureaucratic<br>• Preventative care is not always effective |
| **Opportunites** | **Threats** |
| • New technologies can increase service effectiveness<br>• New therapies can improve treatments<br>• Changes in government policy may strengthen services in the future | • New crises and social problems: climate change, migration<br>• Moves to privatisation<br>• Changes in government policy may lead to break up of services |

Figure 1  A SWOT analysis of health and social care

## Key Question 2: What's your SWOT analysis?

Figure 1 is my own SWOT analysis. Feel free to disagree with it and develop one of your own. You might want to analyse health and social care at a national level, or at a local level for your own area.

- Does your analysis look positive or negative?
- How might your analysis change if, for example, there was a change of government, or a cure for all infectious diseases?

# PREDICTING, CREATING AND DEALING WITH CHANGE: THE PLACE OF RESEARCH

Research and the creation of an evidence base will continue to be central to the effectiveness of health and social care, as far as I can see. With regard to the aim of this book, I want to discuss the relationship between change and research in health and social care in terms of changes as research drivers or as research driven.

## Change as a research driver

Change, or the likelihood of change, can act as a driver for research. In other words, change leads to the development of research projects. Sometimes the change is potentially very positive: it represents an opportunity. Sometimes it's negative, representing a threat.

When change presents us with an opportunity then research will aim to test out ways in which that opportunity can best be taken up. The development of a new drug, for example, drives research projects that seek to ensure it is used effectively in health care. When change presents us with a threat, or at least a potential threat, then research aims to accurately assess the threat, as well as to develop ways of controlling or eliminating it. At the time of writing this chapter the UK media are publishing numerous stories about the threats posed by knife crime and by the use of cannabis. Both of these perceived threats are likely to drive the development of many research projects in health and social care.

Changes that drive research can be planned or unplanned and this in turn will affect how research is managed. Planned changes, whatever their size, are often implemented over a period of months or years. Researchers and funding organisations have advance warning of their appearance and programmes of research can be developed to ensure that studies can be designed and undertaken in appropriate ways and at appropriate times.

Unplanned change catches us out. It is not deliberate, not the result of discussion or development and not amenable to the organisation of a well-structured research programme.

## Research-driven change

Not all health and social care research is a response to change. Some research seeks to create change, either directly or indirectly, through the establishment of new evidence or the creation of new products, procedures or theories. In some cases research projects are established in an attempt to create change in a specific area: to find a cure for malaria, or to create a vaccine against Avian Flu. In other cases researchers might undertake projects without a specific focus, with the hope that their findings might have a use in the future in an as yet unidentified way: so-called 'Blue Skies' research, whose eventual benefits for care might not be known for some years.

# THE INTERNATIONAL NATURE OF HEALTH AND SOCIAL CARE

One of the biggest changes in health and social care, with major implications for research and practice, is its increasing internationalisation, or globalisation. Health care practitioners, especially doctors, have tended to practise internationally for many years (Bach, 2004) but the 'new globalisation' is different and far more extensive. It is likely to affect every reader of this book.

## The globalisation of practice

The global migration of health and social care practitioners is increasing (Diallo, 2004). Some practitioners travel by choice, seeking short periods of experience or education in foreign countries before returning to their home countries to practise for the majority of their careers. Others migrate out of necessity or a desire to improve their working conditions, their social environments or their incomes. The direction of this migration can vary year by year. A few years ago a shortage of health and social care professionals in the UK led to the active recruitment of staff from Spain, the Philippines and elsewhere. In 2007 NHS financial problems are leading to an undersupply of jobs for nurses, therapists and doctors. Health professionals are migrating from the UK to countries such as Australia and the USA, which have acute shortages of qualified staff. Many African and Asian countries are suffering their own shortages of health and social care professionals as their newly-qualified practitioners emigrate to richer nations which can offer better working conditions and higher salaries (Diallo, 2004).

## The globalisation of patients and clients

It's not only practitioners who migrate across the world. Our patients and clients are also migrating in increasing numbers (Koehn, 2004). In the UK the biggest impact on the population in the twenty-first century has been the expansion of the European Community (EC) and the resulting migration from Eastern Europe. Migrants from the expanded EC have moved to the UK for many reasons, but whatever these reasons may be they all have health, social and welfare needs and expectations. UK health and social care practitioners have to develop new skills and knowledge in order to meet these needs.

## Globalisation: its impact on health and social care research and evidence-based practice

Globalisation both challenges and benefits the evidence base for health and social care. The challenge it creates is twofold. Global migration of huge numbers of people changes the health and social care needs of communities and it is doing so in the early twenty-first century at an incredible rate. Global migration of health and social care practitioners changes the skills mix of the care providers within a community and creates the need to reconsider ways of working and professional roles. Evidence for health and social care need can become out of date within a few years or even months. Evidence about care provision can also become outmoded in a short period of time.

Conversely, globalisation of health and social care offers tremendous opportunities for research. In rapidly changing communities and services it becomes impossible to even attempt to justify old-established customs and practices in care provision. Changing populations need responsive, evidence-based, services and so a skilled body of health and social care researchers becomes crucial to effective care delivery.

## WHO WILL BE THE HEALTH AND SOCIAL CARE RESEARCHERS OF THE FUTURE?

The need for health and social care research is not about to disappear. As soon as we answer one question another one arises, as soon as we solve one problem another one presents itself: there is still plenty of work for researchers to do. Indeed, the amount of health and social care research produced annually seems to be increasing. So who will be the health and social care researchers for the twenty-first century?

When I was a student nurse, health and social care researchers were rare. Most health and social care professionals did not require a degree: nurses, social workers, physiotherapists and others qualified at certificate or diploma level and few went on to gain a first degree. Even fewer achieved masters level qualifications and doctorates were almost unheard of. Health and social care research was carried out by doctors, laboratory-based scientists and disciplines such as psychology and sociology. The idea of health and social care research being undertaken by health and social care professionals such as midwives or social workers was slow to gain acceptance. However, as the health and social care professions moved their education programmes into universities and began to insist on graduate practitioners, more and more of these practitioners began to study at higher academic levels. As a result more professionals developed research skills and were able to undertake well-designed research projects. The pool of skilled researchers began to grow rapidly, the researchers started to achieve high-level academic jobs and they began to compete successfully for large research grants.

Although some health and social care researchers worked within the positivist **paradigm**, many of them also started to adopt and develop **naturalistic** research **methodologies** and gradually these methodologies were taken more seriously by funding organisations, practitioners and policy-makers. This in turn helped health and social care researchers to compete with **positivist** researchers from medicine and the bio-medical sciences. The idea that health and social care professionals using naturalistic methodologies can produce high-quality research projects which add to the evidence base is still not universally accepted, but it is greeted with far less scorn and incredulity than it used to be.

But this doesn't mean that every health and social care practitioner must prepare to do research. Research is a specialised activity and to expect all practitioners to undertake research projects is unrealistic. I am strongly in favour of ensuring that health and social care practitioners understand the research process and have the ability to read research reports critically, but ensuring that all health and social care practitioners have the skills to undertake research projects seems unnecessary and, for the foreseeable future, unattainable.

There is certainly a case to be made for preparing more health and social care practitioners to become researchers, but in relatively small numbers. The conclusions of the UK Clinical Research Collaboration (UKCRC, 2006) about the future of nursing research show the scale of this intended preparation clearly.

## KEY CASE 1 – Preparing nurse, midwife and public health nurse researchers

The UKCRC draft report of December 2006 made these recommendations for research training for nurses across the UK.

- *Up to 100* career clinical academic training positions annually, leading to a masters qualification in research.
- *Up to 50* appointments annually (for five years) to three-year full-time or equivalent part-time posts leading to PhD or professional doctorate qualifications.
- *Up to 20* post-doctoral fellowships annually, each lasting three years.
- *Up to 10* senior clinical academic fellowships annually, each lasting three to five years.

There are almost 700,000 nurses, midwives and public health nurses registered in the UK. Even if the UKCRC recommendations were accepted in full this means that a maximum of 180 nurses per year would be undertaking this advanced research training. Nurse researchers will remain a small minority of the profession for many years to come.

## SERVICE USER INVOLVEMENT IN RESEARCH

For me, one of the most interesting questions about the future of health and social care research is the question of service user involvement. Service users, whether they are patients, clients or carers, are routinely recruited as research subjects or participants. Their views and opinions are regularly sought in service evaluation strategies such as satisfaction surveys. But how much more involvement can service users have in the development, design or implementation of research projects?

Figure 2 shows the different levels of service user involvement in research and demonstrates the wide variation in this involvement. Some research methods help to expand the role of the participant to what I've called 'data creator'. The difference between the two relates to the amount of freedom the individual has in providing data and has arisen in particular through the development of new technologies. Data creators have greater freedom to decide what data they provide than do the more usual participants.

| Subject | Providing 'objective' data such as blood samples, responses to quantitative surveys. |
|---|---|
| Participant | Providing 'subjective' data via interviews, diaries, **member checking** and **participant corroboration** |
| Data creator | Active role in collecting data under the direction of researchers |
| Researcher | Involved as an equal partner in design and implementation of research studies |
| Research reviewer | Assessing proposals for projects, sitting on ethics committees, reviewing project reports prior to publication (for example, as a Cochrane Collaboration Lay Reviewer) |
| Research commissioner | Voluntary organisations/user groups commissioning and funding research projects to meet their own specifications |

**Figure 2** Service user involvement in research

In the recent past much of the evidence provided by participants in research was controlled through, for example, the design of questionnaires or interview schedules or the decisions of the researcher undertaking observations. New recording technologies, such as digital cameras or video recorders, enable more of the decision-making to devolve to participants. So, rather than simply interviewing service users about their experiences of disability, homelessness or substance dependency a researcher can ask individuals to record their evidence as and when they wish. Of course, this approach has been available to researchers through the use of written diaries, but the recent explosion in cheap, reliable and easily portable electronic devices makes the method more readily achievable.

Many health and social care researchers appear to be far more open to the idea of service users as researchers than researchers from better-established disciplines. This opening up of the research process is still in its infancy but has huge potential for expansion. The internet and the growing public appetite for its use in 'researching' family trees or holiday destinations is creating a large body of service users who are comfortable with the idea of research and who are developing an interest in this activity within health and social care.

Increasing service user interest is also leading to the involvement of many service users in research review and appraisal. This can involve the appraisal of research proposals submitted to funding bodies, the review of research projects before they are implemented and the review of research papers submitted for publication. Both the Cochrane Collaboration and the Campbell Collaboration encourage active user or 'consumer' involvement in their activities, including the peer reviewing of **systematic reviews** before they are published. Service users, often referred to as 'lay members', also sit on research ethics committees to help in ensuring that projects are ethically sound.

At the highest level of involvement voluntary organisations and user groups are commissioning their own research projects, with some of the wealthier organisations offering large research grants. The ability to commission research studies gives service users the opportunity to control the design, aims and implementation of these projects and to monitor their progress from proposal to dissemination of the findings.

I am a strong supporter of service user involvement in research, but you need to be aware of its potential problems as well as its benefits. The term 'service user involvement' implies that all service users are equally involved, or at least have equal opportunity to be involved, but this is not the case. Involvement in research requires time, effort, knowledge and understanding and a commitment to work with health and social care academics or professionals who often expect too much of their service user colleagues or who can be openly hostile to the users' activities. As a result, service users who take part in these activities may not reflect the broader population of service users: they may be 'unrepresentative'.

Service users involved in research may be more likely to come from academic or professional backgrounds themselves. They may have higher than average incomes, better qualifications and more familiarity with research than the 'typical' service user. They may be older, or less likely to be from an ethnic minority background. For some authors these are major concerns. For others, some service user involvement, even by 'non-representative' individuals, is better than none. My own feeling is that as service user involvement becomes more usual, and people take note of the positive impact it can have, other service users will feel more confident in taking part and the involved user community will become more representative.

## SUMMARY

Health and social care services, practitioners, needs and activities are changing dramatically. I can see no point in the short or medium term at which this change will stop or even slow down. If we hope to be able to match the changing needs of the population with the appropriate changes to service provision then we will need research and reliable evidence more than ever. While the design and implementation of research projects is likely to remain the responsibility of a minority of professionals, every health and social care practitioner needs to be able to make use of evidence and should expect to participate in research, evaluation or audit regularly.

---

## KEY LEARNING POINTS

- Health and social care needs are constantly evolving.
- Health and social care practitioners must be able to respond quickly to ensure that they meet these needs effectively.
- Practitioners' roles and the training, education and abilities needed to fulfil these roles are becoming increasingly complex.
- Globalisation of health and social care is a key issue for the twenty-first century.
- Health and social care practitioners must ensure that they are aware of threats and weaknesses, but should also be ready to capitalise on their strengths and opportunities.

---

## FURTHER READING

Beresford, P and Croft, S (2001) 'Service users' knowledge and the social construction of social work'. *Journal of Social Work*, 1: 295–316

Department of Health (1999) *Patient and public involvement in the new NHS*. London: Department of Health

Department of Health (2007) *Research funding and priorities*. **www.dh.gov.uk/en/Policyandguidance/Researchanddevelopment/A-Z/DH_4069152** (20 June 2007)

Starbuck, WH (2006) *The production of knowledge. The challenge of social science research*. Oxford: Oxford University Press

Telford, R and Faulkner, A (2004) 'Learning about service user involvement in mental health research'. *Journal of Mental Health*, 13: 549–59

United Kingdom Clinical Research Collaboration (2006) *Developing the best research professionals. Qualified graduate nurses: recommendations for preparing and supporting clinical academic nurses of the future*. Draft report

# Glossary

**Bias**: An element of a research study that leads to inaccuracy or misrepresentation in the results. For example, poor selection strategies can lead to a **biased** research sample or the use of leading questions can bias responses in a particular direction. Bias is often accidental, but it can be deliberately introduced as well.

**Blinding:** It is possible to reduce **bias** and improve **reliability** in a study by blinding participants or researchers to some aspect of the research process. This ensures that a key piece of information is not known and therefore does not impact on the way in which the researcher or participant acts. Studies can be double-blind or single-blind. In a **double-blind** study both researcher and participant are blinded. In a **single-blind** study either the researcher or participant will be blinded. In an **unblinded** study neither the researcher nor the participant is blinded.

**Causal relationship**: This means that one variable directly causes a change in another.

**Cohort study**: A research study which follows one or more groups (or cohorts) of subjects over a period of time. This design is often used to investigate the progress of a disease, for example by following a cohort of people with the disease and a cohort who do not have the disease. Cohort studies do not **randomise** subjects.

**Confidence interval**: A range of values for a variable within which the true value of this variable should lie in the population of interest. The interval is usually claimed with 95% confidence, which means that the true value will lie within the given range 95% of the time.

**Control group**: A group of subjects who do not receive the intervention being studied but who resemble the **intervention group** in all other respects.

**Correlation**: A measure of the link between two variables.

**Descriptive statistics**: provide us with information about the data as a whole. They summarise this data and enable the reader to gain a clear idea about the body of results in terms of their similarities and differences. Descriptive statistics normally provide information about three areas: frequency, central tendency and dispersion (Parahoo, 1997). (See also **inferential statistics**.)

**Double-blind**: see **blinding**.

**Ethnography**: A study of a culture or community using a range of fieldwork methods including observation and interviews.

**Experimental**: Where the researchers design an experiment by controlling or altering the subjects of the study or the environment in which it takes place.

**Grounded theory**: A form of research which uses careful coding and classification of data to enable theories to emerge from the information as it is analysed.

**Hypothesis** can be defined as 'a way of proposing a relationship between two or more variables, or factors' (Clifford, 1997, p.92). Wharrad (1998, p.4) describes it as a 'testable proposition about the outcome of an experiment' or an 'educated guess'. A **null hypothesis** predicts no effect, or a negative relationship.

**Inferential statistics**: These are statistics which are used to infer events or actions in a general population based on data from research using a sample population. They enable researchers to predict, or generalise. (See also **descriptive statistics**.)

**Informed consent**: Consent to take part in a research study which is given by an individual based on a clear understanding of the project, its aims and the probable risks or benefits that may result from participation.

**Interpretive**: This **paradigm** sees 'reality' as open to interpretation by those within the environment being studied or by those observing events and actions.

**Intervention group**: A group of subjects who receive the health or social care intervention under study. Also known as the **experimental group**. (See also **control group**.)

**Member checking**: see **participant corroboration**.

**Methodology**: Strictly speaking, 'the study of method'. In modern research this word is used to refer to the ways in which a project can be designed. A methodology is the 'strategy, plan of action, process or design lying behind the choice and use of particular methods and linking the choice and use of methods to the desired outcomes' (Brechin and Sidell, 2000, p.7). (See also **experimental** and **naturalistic**.)

**Naturalistic**: Research where the researchers leave the environment unchanged and do not attempt to manipulate the participants.

**Non-parametric tests**: See **parametric tests**.

**Null hypothesis**: See **hypothesis**.

**Odds ratio (OR)**: A method of measuring the likelihood of an outcome occurring in individuals or groups exposed to a particular variable. If there is no difference between the groups the OR will be 1.0. If a group has an OR of less than 1.0 they are less likely to achieve the outcome, an OR of more than 1.0 means that a group is more likely to achieve the outcome. For example, smokers are more likely to develop lung cancer than non-smokers so the smokers' OR for lung cancer is greater than 1.0.

**Paradigms**: A research paradigm is 'a general theory that informs most scholarship on the operation and outcomes of any particular system of thought and action.' (Entman, 1993, p.56). In other words, it's a system of beliefs and ideas about the best way to find out about the world and, therefore, about research itself. (See also **interpretive** and **positivist**.)

**Parametric tests**: These **inferential** statistical tests can be used only when interval or ratio level measures exist and when data are normally distributed. **Non-parametric tests** can be applied to nominal or ordinal level data and do not need a normal distribution.

**Participant corroboration**: Where interview transcripts are given to interviewees for comment or clarification.

**Phenomenology** is defined by D.W. Smith (2003) as 'the study of "phenomena": appearances of things, or things as they appear in our experience, or the ways we experience things ... Phenomenology studies conscious experience as experienced from the subjective or first person point of view'. This definition focuses on phenomenology's emphasis on the 'lived experience' of individuals, which makes it very attractive to health and social care researchers.

**Pilot study**: A small study carried out to test the methods that are to be used in a larger study. A pilot study is often used to test new methods of data collection, such as questionnaires or interview schedules.

**Positivist**: This **paradigm** sees reality as 'fixed', measurable and predictable and so able to be studied objectively.

**Power calculations** use information about a range of criteria to identify the minimum number of subjects or participants a study needs in order for it to produce statistically significant results.

**Purposive sampling**: A form of sampling in which the research team deliberately select their participants because they have specific characteristics: as Green and Thorogood (2004, p.102) put it, the team are 'explicitly selecting interviewees who it is intended will generate appropriate data'.

**Qualitative data**: Data collected in a non-numerical form (usually as words, but also possibly as images, pictures or objects). Analysis aims to discover underlying meanings or patterns in the data.

**Quantitative data**: Data collected in numerical form so that it can be analysed mathematically or statistically.

**Randomisation**: A method of selecting or allocating participants in a study to minimise the risk of **bias**.

**Randomised controlled trial**: An experimental research design characterised by the random allocation of subjects to each of the **intervention** and **control groups**. This is a standard approach to the study of health and social care interventions, especially drug treatments.

**Reliability**: The extent to which data collection methods will collect the same data on repeated occasions. The more consistently this occurs the more reliable the methods are.

**Research governance**: A system which sets out principles, requirements and standards for research, which defines mechanisms to deliver these principles, requirements and standards, and which improves research and safeguards the public.

**Sampling**: Selecting a proportion of individuals, a sample, from the total population. (See also **purposive sampling**.)

**Single-blind**: See **blinding**.

**Stratification**: In stratified random sampling the total population is subdivided into groups, or strata, according to characteristics that are seen as potentially important to the study.

**Systematic review**: A specialist form of review by which the data from existing research studies on a specific subject can be summarised and re-analysed in order to produce an overview of their results. The overview should create a more reliable set of findings than that provided by the original studies.

**Thematic analysis**: A **qualitative** method used to analyse text (interview transcripts or diary entries, for example) in order to classify this text into different categories or themes.

**Validity**: The extent to which data collection and analysis accurately measure what the researchers intended to measure.

# References

Alcolado, J and Bennett, R (2006) 'Research or audit? Ethical approval for medical student clinical projects'. *Medical Education*, 40: 491

Antle, BJ and Regehr, C (2003) 'Beyond individual rights and freedoms: metaethics in social work research'. *Social Work*, 48: 135–44

Bach, S (2004) 'Migration patterns of physicians and nurses: still the same story?' *Bulletin of the World Health Organization*, 82: 624–5

Benatar, SR (2004) 'Towards progress in resolving dilemmas in international research ethics'. *Journal of Law, Medicine and Ethics*, 32: 574–82

Beresford, P and Croft, S (2001) 'Service users' knowledge and the social construction of social work'. *Journal of Social Work*, 1: 295–316

Bhogal, SK, Teasell, RW, Foley, NC and Speechley, MR (2005) 'The PEDro scale provides a more comprehensive measure of methodological quality than the Jadad Scale in stroke rehabilitation literature'. *Journal of Clinical Epidemiology*, 58: 668–73

Big Lottery Fund (2007) **www.biglotteryfund.org.uk/index/** (29 July 2007)

Bradley, P and Lindsay, B (2001) 'Epilepsy clinics versus general neurology or medical clinics' [update]. *The Cochrane Library*, issue 3

Bradley, PM and Lindsay, B (2007) 'Specialist care for epilepsy and non-epileptic seizures in adults' [protocol]. *The Cochrane Library*, issue 1

Brechin, A and Sidell, M (2000) 'Ways of knowing'; in Gomm, R and Davies, C (eds) *Using evidence in health and social care*. London: Open University/Sage

Burke Johnson, R and Onwuegbuzie, AJ (2004) 'Mixed methods research: a research paradigm whose time has come'. *Educational Researcher*, 33: 14–26

Burns, N and Grove, SK (1999) *Understanding nursing research* (2nd edn). Philadelphia: WB Saunders

Butler, I (2002) 'A code of ethics for social work and social care research'. *British Journal of Social Work*, 32: 239–48

Caplin, DA, Rao, JK, Filloux, F, Bale, JF and Van Orman, C (2006) 'Development of performance indicators for the primary care management of pediatric epilepsy: expert consensus recommendations based on the available evidence'. *Epilepsia*, 47: 2011–2019

Chapman, S and Shatenstein, S (2001) 'The ethics of the cash register: taking tobacco research dollars'. *Tobacco Control*, 10: 1–2

Chronic Poverty Research Centre (undated) *Methods toolbox: overarching issues.* **www.chronicpoverty.org/CPToolbox/Overarchingissues.htm** (13 June 2007)

Clancy, CM and Cronin, K (2005) 'Evidence-based decision making: global evidence, local decisions'. *Health Affairs*, 24: 151–62

Clifford, C (1997) *Nursing and health care research* (2nd edn). London: Prentice Hall

Coggon, D, Rose, G and Barker, DJP (1993) *Epidemiology for the uninitiated* (3rd edn). London: BMJ Publishing Group

Coghlan, D and Brannick, T (2005) *Doing action research in your own organization* (2nd edn). London: Sage

Concato, J, Shah, N and Horwitz, RI (2000) 'Randomized, controlled trials, observational studies and the hierarchy of research designs'. *New England Journal of Medicine*, 342: 1887–92

COREC Ethics Consultation E-Group (2006) *Differentiating audit, service evaluation and research.* **www.nres.npsa.nhs.uk/applicants/help/guidance.htm#audit** (20 June 2007)

Coren, E, Patterson, J, Astin, M and Abbott, J (2003) 'Home-based support for socially disadvantaged mothers. (Protocol)'. *Cochrane Database of Systematic Reviews*, issue 1

Cornish, K (1998) *Trent focus for research and development in primary health care: an introduction to using statistics in research.* Nottingham: Trent Focus

Coupland, H and Maher, L (2005) 'Clients or colleagues? Reflections on the process of participatory action research with young injecting drug users'. *The International Journal of Drug Policy*, 16: 191–8

Department of Health (1999) *Patient and public involvement in the new NHS.* London: Department of Health

Department of Health (2005) *Research governance framework for health and social care.* London: Department of Health

Department of Health (2007) *Research funding and priorities.* **www.dh.gov.uk/en/Policyandguidance/Researchanddevelopment/A-Z/DH_4069152** (20 June 2007)

Diallo, K (2004) 'Data on the migration of health-care workers: sources, uses, and challenges'. *Bulletin of the World Health Organization*, 82: 601–7

Diaper, G (1990) 'The Hawthorne Effect: a fresh examination'. *Educational Studies*, 16: 261–8

Entman, RM (1993) 'Framing: toward clarification of a fractured paradigm'. *Journal of Communication*, 43: 51–8

EPOC (2002) The data collection checklist. **www.epoc.uottawa.ca/tools.htm** (20 June 2007)

Fouché, G (2006) 'Respected Norwegian scientist faked study on oral cancer'. *Guardian*, 16 January

Fox, M, Martin, P and Green, G (2007) *Doing practitioner research.* London: Sage

Gilgun, JF (2005) 'The four cornerstones of evidence-based practice in social work'. *Research on Social Work Practice*, 15: 52–61

Gomm, R and Davies, C (2000) (eds) *Using evidence in health and social care.* London: Open University/Sage

Gould, D (1994) 'Writing literature reviews'. *Nurse Researcher*, 2: 13–23

Grbich, C (2007) *Qualitative data analysis. An introduction.* London: Sage

Green, J and Thorogood, N (2004) *Qualitative methods for health research.* London: Sage

Haggerty, KD (2004) 'Ethics creep: governing social science research in the name of ethics'. *Qualitative Sociology*, 27: 391–414

Hanley, T (2006) 'Mick Cooper. Counselling in schools project: evaluation report'. *Counselling and Psychotherapy Research*, 6: 150–1

Hart, E, Lymbery, M and Gladman, JRF (2005) 'Away from home: an ethnographic study of a transitional rehabilitation scheme for older people in the UK'. *Social Science and Medicine*, 60: 1241–50

Hayes, J (2007) *The theory and practice of change management.* New York: Palgrave Macmillan

Hearnshaw, H (2004) 'Comparison of requirements of research ethics committees in 11 European countries for a non-invasive interventional study'. *British Medical Journal*, 328: 140–1

HERO (1999) *Guidance on Submissions.* RAE 2/99. **www.hero.ac.uk/rae/niss/2_99.html** (8 June 2007)

Holbeche, l (2006) *Understanding change: theory, implementation and success.* Oxford: Elsevier Butterworth Heinemann

Holden, JD (2001) 'Hawthorne effects and research into professional practice'. *Journal of Evaluation in Clinical Practice*, 7: 65–70

Holliday, A (2007) *Doing and writing qualitative research* (2nd edn). London: Sage

Horton, R (2006a) 'Expression of concern: non-steroidal anti-inflammatory drugs and the risk of oral cancer'. *The Lancet*, 367: 196

Horton, R (2006b) 'Retraction – non-steroidal anti-inflammatory drugs and the risk of oral cancer; a nested case-control study'. *The Lancet*, 367: 382

Humphries, B (2003) 'What *else* counts as evidence in evidence-based social work?' *Social Work Education*, 22: 81–91

Jamtvedt, G, Young, JM, Kristoffersen, DT, O'Brien, MA and Oxman, AD (2006) 'Audit and feedback: effects on professional practice and health care outcomes'. *Cochrane Database of Systematic Reviews*, issue 2

Jones, GR (2007) *Organizational theory, design and change.* New Jersey: Pearson Prentice Hall

Katrak, P, Bialocerkowski, AE, Massy-Westropp, N, Saravana Kumar, VS and Grimmer, KA (2004) 'A systematic review of the content of critical appraisal tools'. *BMC Medical Research Methodology*, 4: 22. **www.biomedcentral.com/1471-2288/4/22** (7 March 2007)

Koehn, PH (2004) 'Global politics and multinational health-care encounters: assessing the role of transnational competence'. *EcoHealth*, 1: 69–85

Kouvonen, A and Lintonen, T (2002) 'Adolescent part-time work and heavy drinking in Finland'. *Addiction*, 97: 311–18

Krauss, SE (2005) 'Research paradigms and meaning making: a primer'. *The Qualitative Report*, 10: 758–70

Lanoe, N (2002) *Ogier's reading research* (3rd edn). London: Bailliére Tindall

Lee, P (2006) 'Understanding some naturalistic research methodologies'. *Paediatric Nursing*, 18: 44–6

Lincoln, YS and Guba, EG (1985) *Naturalistic inquiry*. London: Sage

Lindsay, B (2007) '"Lawrence Blaine is unwell": a web-based international "community of practice" to engage nursing students in the planning and delivery of health care', in Remenyi, D (ed) *ICEL 2007 2nd International Conference on E-Learning* (Conference Proceedings). Reading: Academic Conferences International

Lindsay, B, Cooper, N and McDonald, H (2001) *Nursing research output study*. Norwich: School of Nursing and Midwifery, University of East Anglia

McCarthy, M (2000) 'An evaluative research study of a specialist women's refuge'. *Journal of Adult Protection*, 2: 29–40

Maio, G (2002) 'The cultural specificity of research ethics – or why ethical debate in France is different'. *Journal of Medical Ethics*, 28: 147–50

Maltby, J, Day, L and Williams, G (2007) *Introduction to statistics for nurses*. Harlow: Pearson Education

Malterud, K (2001) 'Qualitative research: standards, challenges, and guidelines'. *The Lancet*, 358: 483–88

Margetts, JK, Le Couteur, A and Croom, S (2006) 'Families in a state of flux: the experience of grandparents in autism spectrum disorder'. *Child: Care, Health and Development*, 32: 565–74

Mathers, N and Huang, YC (1998) 'Evaluating methods for analyzing data in published research', in Crookes, P and Davies, S (eds) *Research into practice. Essential skills for reading and applying research in nursing and health care*. London: Baillière Tindall

Medical Research Council (2005) *Good research practice. MRC ethics series*. London: MRC

Medical Research Council (2006) *MRC annual report and accounts* 2005/06. London: MRC

Miles, MB and Huberman, AM (1994) *Qualitative data analysis: an expanded sourcebook*. (2nd edn). Thousand Oaks: Sage

Miller, FG (2004) 'Research ethics and misguided moral intuition'. *Journal of Law, Medicine and Ethics*, 32: 111–6

Morrison, J (2003) 'ABC of learning and teaching in medicine: evaluation'. *British Medical Journal*, 326: 385–7

National Health and Medical Research Council of Australia (1999) *National statement on ethical conduct in research involving humans*. **www.nhmrc.gov.au/publications/synopses/_files/e35.pdf** (6 March 2007)

National Research Ethics Service (2007) **www.nres.npsa.nhs.uk/** (29 July 2007)

National Statistics (2006) **www.statistics.gov.uk/** (29 July 2007)

Neale, J, Allen, D and Coombes, L (2005) 'Qualitative research methods within the addictions'. *Addiction*, 100:1584–93

Needham, G (2000) 'Research and practice: making a difference', in Gomm, R and Davies, C (eds) *Using evidence in health and social care*. London: Open University/Sage

Ogier, ME (1998) *Reading research* (2nd edn). London: Baillière Tindall

Onwuegbuzie, AJ and Leech, NL (2005) 'Taking the 'Q' out of research: teaching research methodology courses without the divide between quantitative and qualitative paradigms'. *Quality and Quantity*, 39: 267–96

Parahoo, K (1997) *Nursing research: principles, process and issues* Basingstoke: Macmillan

Parahoo K (2006) *Nursing research: principles, process and issues* (2nd edn). London: Palgrave Macmillan

Parry, CJ and Lindsay, WR (2003) 'Impulsiveness as a factor in sexual offending by people with mild intellectual disability'. *Journal of Intellectual Disability Research*, 47:1: 81–90

Paterson, C, Allen, J.A, Browning, M, Barlow, G and Ewings, P (2005) 'A pilot study of therapeutic massage for people with Parkinson's disease: the added value of user involvement'. *Complementary Therapies in Clinical Practice*, 11: 161–71

Prideaux, D and Rogers, W (2006) 'Audit or research: the ethics of publication'. *Medical Education*, 40: 497–99

Public Health Resource Unit (2006) *Critical appraisal tools.* **www.phru.nhs.uk/casp/critical_appraisal_tools.htm** (7 March 2007)

Rycroft-Malone, J, Seers, K, Titchen, A, Harvey, G, Kitson, A and McCormack, B (2004) 'What counts as evidence in evidence-based practice?' *Journal of Advanced Nursing*, 47: 81–90

Sackett, DL, Richardson, WS, Rosenberg, W and Haynes RB (1997) *Evidence based medicine. How to practice and teach EBM.* Edinburgh: Churchill Livingstone

Sanders, RM (2003) 'Medical research ethics committees and social work research: a hurdle too far?' *Social Work Education*, 22: 113–14

Shaw, I.F (2003) 'Ethics in qualitative research and evaluation'. *Journal of Social Work*, 3: 9–29

Shaw, I (2005) 'Practitioner research: evidence or critique?' *British Journal of Social Work*, 35: 1231–48

Smith, DW (2003) 'Phenomenology'. *Stanford encyclopedia of philosophy.* **http://plato.stanford.edu/entries/phenomenology/** (26 June 2007)

Smith, GCS and Pell, JP (2003) 'Parachute use to prevent death and major trauma related to gravitational challenge: systematic review of randomised controlled trials'. *British Medical Journal*, 327: 1459–61

Smith, KL, Soriano, TA and Boal, J (2007) 'Brief communication: national quality-of-care standards in home-based primary care'. *Annals of Internal Medicine*, 146: 188–92

Starbuck, WH (2006) *The production of knowledge. The challenge of social science research*. Oxford: Oxford University Press

Stewart, S, Harvey, I, Poland, F, Lloyd-Smith, W, Mugford, M and Flood, C (2005) 'Are occupational therapists more effective than social workers when assessing frail older people? Results of CAMELOT, a randomised controlled trial'. *Age and Ageing*, 34: 41–6

Sudbø, J, Lee, JJ, Lippman, SM, Mork, J, Sagen, S, Flatner, N, Ristimaki, A, Sudbø, A, Mao, L, Zhou, X, Kildal, W, Evensen, JF, Reith, A and Dannenberg, AJ (2005) 'Non-steroidal anti-inflammatory drugs and the risk of oral cancer: a nested case-control study'. *The Lancet*, 366: 1359–66

Telford, R and Faulkner, A (2004) 'Learning about service user involvement in mental health research'. *Journal of Mental Health*, 13: 549–59

Thomson, AM (1998) 'Recognizing research processes in research-based literature', in Crookes, PA and Davies, S (eds) *Research into practice*. Edinburgh: Baillière Tindall

United Kingdom Clinical Research Collaboration (2006) *Developing the best research professionals. Qualified graduate nurses: recommendations for preparing and supporting clinical academic nurses of the future*. Draft report

Wakefield, AJ, Murch, SH, Anthony, A, Linnell, J, Casson, DM, Malik, M, Berelowitz, M, Dhillon, AP, Thomson, MA, Harvey, P, Valentine, A, Davies, SE and Walker-Smith, JA (1998) 'Ileal-lymphoid-nodular hyperplasia, non-specific colitis, and pervasive developmental disorder in children'. *The Lancet*, 351: 637–41

Waldman, J (2005) 'Using evaluative research to support practitioners and service users in undertaking reflective writing for public dissemination'. *British Journal of Social Work* 35: 975–81.

Wharrad, H (1998) *Trent focus for research and development in primary health care: an introduction to experimental designs*. Nottingham: Trent Focus

Whitaker, S and Hirst, D (2002) 'Correlational analysis of challenging behaviours'. *British Journal of Learning Disabilities*, 30: 28–31

Wilson, K, Fyson, R and Newstone, S (2007) 'Foster fathers: their experiences and contributions to fostering'. *Child and Family Social Work*, 12: 22–31

World Medical Association (2004) *Declaration of Helsinki. World Medical Association*. **www.wma.net/e/policy/pdf/17c.pdf** (February 2007)

Wright, CM, Callum, J, Birks, E and Jarvis, S (1998) 'Effect of community based management in failure to thrive: randomised controlled trial'. *British Medical Journal*, 317: 571–4

Yin, RK (2003) *Case study research design and methods. Applied social research methods series* volume 5. Thousand Oaks: Sage

# Index

individual, primacy of 51–2
inferential statistics 81
informed consent 35, 54, 63–4
internationalisation 135–6
internet dissemination 96
interpretive paradigm 3, 29, 31, 62,
    73, 89, 115
intervention group 68, 123
interviews 66–7

Jamtvedt, G 124

Katrak, P 25
knowledge from local context 123
Kouvonen, A 9

Lee, P 30
Leech, NL 73, 74
limitations
    accuracy 89–91, 98
    honesty 90–1
    and understanding 87–9, 91
Lincoln, YS 73, 85
Lindsay, WR 10
Lintonen, T 9
literature review
    age of research 18
    aims 13
    appraisal tools 25
    backgrounds of researchers 16
    context 14–17
    criteria 19
    critical approach 18
    databases *see* databases
    evaluation 24–5
    existing research 14–15
    funding amount 16
    grey literature 24
    as justification 18
    library searches 23
    methods 17
    provenance 16
    stages 19
    strategy 19–20
    summary 26

Maher, L 118
Margetts, JK 9
marketing 114
mass media 114
maximum variation sampling 61
mean 78–9
measurement scales 75–6

median 78
member checking 57
methodologies 29, 31, 116
methods 30, 31, 35–7
Miles, MB 83
mode 78
moral relativism 51
Morrison, J 124

naturalistic methodology 33–5, 39,
    105, 116, 137
Needham, G 113
non-parametric tests 80
non-steroidal anti-inflammatory drugs
    (NSAIDs) 91
Nuremburg code 49

observation 67
Onwuegbuzie, AJ 73, 74
opportunistic sampling 61

paradigms 3, 29, 31–2, 62, 73–4
parametric tests 80
Parry, CJ 10
participants
    corroboration 57
    payments 47, 64
    recruitment issues 57
    safety 54
participatory action research (PAR) 118
passive dissemination 113
Paterson, C 59, 62
PEDro Scale 105
Pell, JP 108
performance management 114
phenomenology 8, 33, 62, 66–7
physiological data 65
pilot study 48
positivist hierarchy 39
positivist paradigm 3, 29, 31–2, 62,
    74, 115, 137
power calculations 62
practice
    *see also* change management;
        evidence-based practice
    globalisation 136
practitioner research 115–16, 118–19
Prideaux, D 124
primacy of the individual 51
professional pressures 40
proformas 66
psychological data 65
purposive sampling 61